First Nations Australian Theatre for Health Equity

Sarah Woodland • Kamarra Bell-Wykes

First Nations Australian Theatre for Health Equity

Healing Stories

palgrave
macmillan

Sarah Woodland
University of Melbourne
Melbourne, VIC, Australia

Kamarra Bell-Wykes
Independent Artist, Melbourne, VIC
Australia

ISBN 978-3-031-65505-0 ISBN 978-3-031-65506-7 (eBook)
https://doi.org/10.1007/978-3-031-65506-7

Cover illustration: Pi_Mo_09 Pattern © Melisa Hasan

This Palgrave Macmillan imprint is published by the registered company Springer Nature Switzerland AG.
The registered company address is: Gewerbestrasse 11, 6330 Cham, Switzerland

Foreword

I was humbled and honoured to be asked to write this foreword for Kamarra and Sarah on this timely review of Kamarra's canon of "applied" theatre, her role to date in that genre, and how it will impact their future work. Their kind offer made me instantly reflect on when I was involved in establishing Ilbijerri Theatre Company, in 1990, and I approached the local Aboriginal Legal Service to get assistance with Ilbijerri's incorporation as a then State-Based Co-operative. The lawyer said I needed to write a mission statement. I came up with what I considered the rather idealistic following statement:

> *Ilbijerri will provide a creative platform for the Victorian Aboriginal community to express their issues and their concerns to themselves and the wider community.*

My first priority as an artist has been to attract my people to the theatre by writing about issues pertinent to us, reflecting from our eyes, and ultimately resolved by us. I have always found it dryly amusing that historically, as First Nations playwrights, we were expected to educate the invaders about their wrongdoing and the effects this has had on us in order to be looked upon kindly by the coloniser. The work about us had to be written for them.

Cultural practices and concepts I have grown up with, such as yarning, relational accountability, strength-based attitude, and positionality, are now acknowledged as important, legitimate, and vital in the development of global First Nations applied theatre and embedded in academic epistemologies far and wide.

The contribution of First Nations artists to their mainstream counterparts and theatres is rarely evaluated, and the influence we have had on even the most successful non-First Nations Australian artists and companies is rarely discussed. My contention is that it is precisely this lack of reflection that contributes to an undermining of our worth to the whole of the arts industry in this country.

Kamarra Bell-Wykes' contribution to date as a playwright and play maker is a powerful statement, her canon of Health education works not only unique but ground-breaking, artistically successful, and inspiring. Kamarra's independent practice and, more recently, her work with collective A Daylight Connection is equally brilliant and capturing the highest accolades.

Dr Sarah Woodland's own history of artistic work has also greatly contributed to the development of Australian applied theatre. This book represents the opportunity to bring together two sharply tuned fine minds to evaluate and honour Kamarra's legacy to date and highlight First Nations communities' ongoing contribution to health education theatre in this country.

The endgame of their research is to highlight the importance of culturally led, culturally focused, and culturally safe practices both in creative development and performance of theatre for health education. This book also represents a gift to the mainstream artistic and health industries. The lessons being shared within these pages, if taken on board, will not only assist in improving applied theatre practice but also inform the potential funders and practitioners within the health industry. I take this opportunity as a Blak playmaker to honour and thank Kamarra and Sarah for all their brilliance to date, and for the reader to listen to the truth in these pages, as in the end they are a gift for us to share with all our communities.

Nothing about us without us.

John Harding

September 2023

It really was a happy circumstance that, in between vetting calls from people wanting Aboriginal names for their dogs/cats/lizards or support with an Aboriginal character written by a non-Aboriginal author that the then Ilbijerri General Manager, Kim Kruger, took seriously a call from an employee from the (then) Victorian Department of Health and Human

Services (DHHS) wanting to address the alarming and growing rates of hepatitis C within Victorian Aboriginal communities. I now pay homage to that DHHS worker, Bronwyn Kaaden, who, thinking outside the box, reached out to community through Ilbijerri to find solutions, or at least to get the word out that this was an issue that we could do something about. Ilbijerri then reached out to our peak Victorian Aboriginal Health organisation VACCHO along with Hepatitis Victoria for their expertise and knowledge, thus beginning a long and prosperous partnership.

Following the line of happenstance, Ilbijerri was also incredibly lucky to have at hand an Aboriginal playwright who, despite the incredibly prescriptive nature of the brief, was able to deliver an amazing piece of theatre that was first and foremost entertaining, as well as delivering a powerful message of hope and power. Kamarra Bell-Wykes had the smarts, talent, and vision back in 2004 to take on this huge responsibility and, almost two decades on, is still delivering, getting more masterful and daring in her theatre practice of being entertaining, challenging, and holding up a mirror to impact and advocate for change.

I must admit I was a bit alarmed that Ilbijerri later labelled these "health message" plays under the banner of "Social Impact," as to my mind, all Ilbijerri productions follow this mantra. It is at the heart of what meaningful Aboriginal theatre is about—to resonate and cater first and foremost to us because it is by us. Kamarra's extraordinary body of work does just this and I am so excited that we can all now witness this in *First Nations Theatre for Health Equity: Healing Stories.*

Kylie Belling
September 2023

Melbourne, VIC, Australia
September 2023

John Harding
Kylie Belling

Acknowledgements

This book was completed with the support of Ilbijerri Theatre Company and its leadership team, Rachael Maza AO (Artistic Director and Co-CEO) and Angela Flynn (Executive Director and Co-CEO). The study informing the book was undertaken with support and funding from the University of Melbourne, Faculty of Fine Arts and Music and approval from the University of Melbourne's Human Research Ethics Committee (ethics ID 14332). We would like to thank Ilbijerri's previous Senior Producer, Kim Bennett, and Associate Producer, Lauren Sheree, for their support in establishing the research partnership, and current Social Impact Producer, Laura Harris, for her tireless work in developing and nurturing the partnership further. We would also like to thank the past practitioners who kindly shared their insights in interviews for the research and to acknowledge the excellent work of Dr Molly McPhee (Goldsmiths University of London) for conducting a literature review. Full acknowledgement of the artists and contributors to Ilbijerri's Social Impact stream will feature through the volume and are listed in the conclusion, however, we acknowledge that this work builds on millennia of important cultural practice, knowledge generation, and healing business undertaken by First Nations peoples across what is now known as Australia. The research was conducted and the book was produced on the unceded lands of the Boonwurrung and Wurundjeri Woi-Wurrung peoples of the Kulin Nations and the Yuggera and Turrbul peoples. We acknowledge Elders past and present on those lands, and everywhere, in leading the way in this vital cultural work focused on education and wellbeing for First Nations communities.

Contents

List of Figures

List of Tables

CHAPTER 1

Introduction

Abstract This book investigates a series of health education plays produced by Australia's Ilbijerri Theatre Company and led by Butchulla and Yuggera theatre maker Kamarra Bell-Wykes from 2005 to 2019. Over this period, Ilbijerri produced and toured five works that provided education around key health issues facing Aboriginal and Torres Strait Islander peoples and communities: *Chopped Liver* (2006–2009; 2017), *Body Armour* (2010–2013) and *Viral – Are You the Cure?* (2018/2019)—also known as the Hepatitis C Trilogy—all deal with hepatitis C transmission, management, and treatment; *North West of Nowhere* (2014–2016) addresses sexual health and healthy relationships; and *Scar Trees* (2019) addresses family violence. Through a comprehensive study, we critically examine these works, while also documenting and acknowledging their important legacy and contribution to theatre for health promotion and education. This chapter describes the research context, methods, and sources of data, as well as our analytical approach informing the study. We introduce how the works operate at the interface between traditional and contemporary First Nations knowledges and performance practices and non-Indigenous approaches to performing arts, education, and wellbeing, also reflecting the cross-cultural relationality and knowledge sharing between we two authors. The chapter concludes with an overview of how the book is organised.

S. Woodland, K. Bell-Wykes, *First Nations Australian Theatre for Health Equity*, https://doi.org/10.1007/978-3-031-65506-7_1

Keywords First Nations theatre • Theatre in education • Applied theatre • Arts and health • Theatre for health education

Ilbijerri Theatre Company is Australia's longest established First Nations[1] theatre company, with a thirty-plus-year legacy of producing highly successful productions that showcase Aboriginal and Torres Strait Islander narratives to broad critical acclaim. Since 2005, Ilbijerri has produced and toured works that provide education and messaging around key health issues facing Aboriginal and Torres Strait Islander peoples and communities, with the majority of these being led by award-winning playwright and theatre maker Kamarra Bell-Wykes (co-author). Since their inception, these works have been commissioned and funded by the state of Victoria's Department of Health, with additional funding and support from various other government and philanthropic sources depending on the health concerns being addressed. The works have specifically (although not exclusively) targeted Aboriginal and Torres Strait Islander audiences in diverse settings, such as prisons, rehabilitation centres, schools, health services, and communities throughout Victoria and nationally. *Chopped Liver* (2006–2009; 2017), *Body Armour* (2010–2013) and *Viral – Are You the Cure?* (2018/2019)—also known as the Hepatitis C Trilogy—all deal with hepatitis C transmission, management, and treatment; *North West of Nowhere* (2014–2016) addresses sexual health and healthy relationships; and *Scar Trees* (2019) addresses family violence.[2] A subsequent work, *Goodbye Aunty Flo* (2023–), written and directed by Nazaree Dickerson,

[1] For this book, we adopt the terms "First Nations" and "Aboriginal and/or Torres Strait Islander" to refer to the First Peoples of so-called Australia. Wherever possible, we identify the specific language groups of individuals. First Nations is a commonly used collective term for the team and stakeholders involved in the research and reflects usage by the wider arts sector in Australia. We also adopt the term "Indigenous," respecting that this collective term refers to the original peoples of Canada and their descendants, and is also used in Australia to refer to Indigenous ways of knowing, being, and doing in research and practice.

[2] Kamarra's scripts for *Chopped Liver* (2018a), *North West of Nowhere* (2018b), and *Body Armour* (2018c) have all since been published by the Australian Script Centre (AustralianPlays.org). Excerpts from the unpublished scripts for *Viral* (written by Maryanne Sam) and *Scar Trees* (which Kamarra adapted from the original script by Declan Furber Gillick) have been included with permission from those writers. We include these in the reference list, however, for ease of reading, we have elected to omit in-text citation details for the plays throughout the remainder of the volume (with the exception of directly quoted excerpts from the published plays).

addresses menopause for Aboriginal and Torres Strait Islander women and falls outside the scope of our study. The works were supported by a reference group of health professionals from organisations such as the Victorian Department of Health, the Victorian Aboriginal Community Controlled Health Organisation (VACCHO) and Hepatitis C Victoria, who provided information and advice on the content of the plays, with local Aboriginal Community Controlled Health Organisations (ACCHOs) being on hand at performances to provide health advice to attendees. These works have to date reached over 26,000 audience members and won numerous awards, including an Indigenous Community Justice Award (2008), a Victorian Public Healthcare Award (2008), and a Creative Partnerships Australia Arts and Health Award (2013). The performances have left lasting impacts in communities, with anecdotal reports of audience members still talking about them years later.

The purpose of this book is to document and honour the legacy of this extremely valuable body of work, which has been somewhat quietly achieving outcomes for Ilbijerri and communities across the country in the background of the company's more high-profile mainstage productions. While there has been some recognition, documentation, and evaluation of works over the years, we undertook a comprehensive study drawing previous resources together and conducting additional research of our own to investigate the approaches used and outcomes achieved. Importantly, this draws on the unique perspective of co-author Kamarra, who has been instrumental in realising the plays through her various roles, first as writer and later as dramaturg, facilitator, and director. We believe that an examination of the creative processes involved in making these works, their cultural, aesthetic, and educational qualities, and their impacts on communities and audiences will provide important insights into theatre for health promotion and education globally, as articulated through a unique First Nations Australian perspective.

The original study also had another important focus. While the health education performances have been extremely engaging for audiences and have provided health information in effective and dynamic ways (as will be revealed in subsequent chapters), the works discussed here were largely created and toured using a more conventional approach— researched and written by a commissioned playwright, rehearsed by a team of professional actors, and then toured into communities. Performances were followed by an audience question-and-answer (Q&A) and yarning circle,[3] and then the touring party moved on. On some occasions, there was a certain degree of community engagement through workshopping ideas for the performances, as will be discussed later. Ultimately, the performances adopted a "fly in-fly out" approach to health education and messaging through theatre. Based on her longstanding experience of leading these works and the findings from this study, Kamarra recently identified a need to explore a more community-engaged, participatory approach that would build capacity in communities and generate lasting health and wellbeing outcomes. This led to the development of *The Score*, a work focused on sexual health, respectful relationships, and sexually transmissible infections (STIs) for Aboriginal and Torres Strait Islander young people that involves engaging community members from the ground up, from the seed of the project to the creation, performance, and touring of the work. At the time of writing, *The Score* is still being developed and refined (in collaboration with co-author Sarah), but our study of previous approaches to the health education works discussed in this book provided the foundational 'looking back' that was necessary for developing *The Score*.

Before we introduce further details about the methods and content of our study, we must first acknowledge our positionality as authors and collaborators. As identified by scholars such as Thorner et al. (2018) and Syron (2021), this is crucial to engaging in ethical, respectful, and relationally grounded cross-cultural practice and research. Given the prominence of yarning throughout all aspects of this project, we present certain passages in this volume as verbatim text, recorded during research discussions and interviews and transcribed later. In some cases, we have edited these for sense or to eliminate unnecessary words or conversational tangents. This approach is now gaining traction in scholarly research as a legitimate form of knowledge generation and reporting that recognises the strong oral traditions within Aboriginal and Torres Strait Islander cultures and privileges First Nations' ways of knowing, being, and doing (see Barlo et al. 2021; Thorner et al. 2018; Woodland et al. 2023). Positionality, in an Aboriginal and Torres Strait Islander yarning context, usually follows

[3] A "yarning circle" refers to a group discussion where each person speaks in turn. Yarning is a complex practice in Aboriginal and Torres Strait Islander cultures that reflects and maintains social relations and facilitates knowledge creation and transmission (see Barlo et al. 2021, and Bessarab and Ng'andu 2010). We centre yarning throughout this book in different ways as integral to all aspects of creating, researching, and reporting on the health education works under discussion.

the dramaturgy of 'who are you, and where are you from?' And in cases where there is a project or cross-cultural collaboration being introduced, 'how did we get here?'

Kamarra: I am descendant of the Yuggera and Butchulla people of south-east Queensland; and then on my father's side, we have a mix of different types of colonial or settler blood. The term that I've learned more recently, and how I now think about myself, is a member of the Aboriginal diaspora. I was born in Naarm (Melbourne), Kulin Country but I was moved to Mparntwe (Alice Springs), Arrernte Country by the time I was three months old, and then spent most of my primary school years moving every six months or so to different Aboriginal communities or to cities, kind of following my Mum around (who was the acclaimed Aboriginal linguist Jeanie Bell) or going to my Dad, who also lived a bit 'off-grid.' So I had a pretty transient childhood, but Melbourne seems to be the place where I have always come back to—predominantly because of the arts, because it's where there's always been more of a stable foundation, even though my mother's family are all up in Queensland and from Cherbourg and K'gari (Fraser Island). I didn't really get to put my roots down in those places as much as I would have liked, and I suppose I have a sense of that that gap sometimes of feeling like I've lived off Country for a good part of my life.

I have started to embrace the fact that my transient lifestyle growing up has given me an opportunity to really observe and experience and be a part of a lot of different Mobs[4] in a lot of different environments. This has given me an open perspective on what lived experience can be. But also combined with the fact that growing up, I also ran the streets quite a bit, and got into quite a bit of trouble, and knocked around with a lot of different Mobs that were doing the 'wrong thing', and people living with addiction, and struggling with addictions myself, and being a young single parent. But through my Mum, I was also exposed to a lot of political movements as a kid as well. I think all these things have contributed to the kind of perspective I have, which I think very much is about having a lot of compas-

[4] "Mob" is a term widely used in Aboriginal and Torres Strait Islander cultures for groups of people associated with a particular family/kinship network, place, country, or cultural group.

sion for the underdog, and for people who feel excluded from society or feel like they have fallen between the cracks, or they don't really belong. This has really helped me to work in spaces and speak to people and create work that really speaks to the truth of people's various lived experiences. I think it's one of the reasons why I'm a good artist, and why I work well in community. Because I meet people where they are, and I think that those kind of voices of the downtrodden are the most interesting. I think witnessing my mother's language work in prisons and visiting family in jail also planted a seed in me. Seeing so many of our community inside and how grateful they were for something, for anything, for knowledge, to know someone actually gave a shit. You've haven't experienced theatre until you watch it with a prison audience. There's nothing like it.

When I first got asked to write *Chopped Liver*, it was a bit of a shock to my system because I had hep C and I hadn't told anyone. But I would have to say that my lived experience was absolutely an essential part of me being able to write the first play with as much heart and truth in it because the play became about the emotional truth of living with hep C more than anything, and that came from my own experiences. When I wrote *Chopped Liver*, I was young myself, and I don't think I fully understood the journey was about to embark on or how significant writing that work really was in terms of my own journey of hep C awareness. After spending seven years in the Northern Territory and getting my education degree at Bachelor institute, studying, and living with Mob from all over Australia, I returned to Melbourne and Ilbijerri to build their education program bringing with me new skills, knowledge and determination, not realising this was just another step in this ongoing social impact journey—that I was only realising how significant this work actually was.

It wasn't until I started directing the works that I really had license to take creative ownership over the works as well. That started to shift my thinking about them as a writer. I have always been taught the culture at certain companies where you only have power while you're writing the script, and then you hand it over, and that's it, you don't get any voice anymore. But once I started directing them, I was like, "Okay, I'm driving the ship now." Writing and performance have always been a magical escape for me. A place where reality is transformed, and experience transported. Where you get to see the world through someone else's eyes and express the things you can't usually verbalise. To be honest creative expression has probably saved my life more than once; given me something to hold onto when there was nothing else. That's what I want to share with Mob.

Sarah: I am a woman with Anglo-European settler ancestry from England, Ireland, Wales, and Germany. I was born in 1970s South Africa, where my Anglo-English mother and Anglo-Australian father lived at the time, very briefly witnessing the terrible injustices of the apartheid era before moving first to Bolivia and then to Australia. I think these early experiences of other cultures and power struggles contributed to my lifelong interest in pursuing ideals of social justice. From the age of five, I grew up on unceded Yuggera, Turrbul Country in Meanjin (Brisbane), which I still feel is my home. Currently, I live and work on the Boonwurrung and Wurundjeri Woiwurrung Country of the Eastern Kulin Nations (south side of Melbourne), but I return to Brisbane to be with family and friends whenever I can. For nearly 30 years, my professional life has been focused on applied theatre and community engaged participatory arts as a practitioner and researcher. In my undergraduate drama degree at Queensland University of Technology, I was exposed to the potential for educational and community-based theatre and was hooked. On graduating, I formed an educational theatre company with some mates and went from there. A formative experience for me was joining Geese Theatre Company in the UK, which works in prisons, criminal justice settings, and criminalised communities. With Geese, I learned so much about performance, facilitation, and the potential for theatre to engender a sense of freedom in even the most oppressive environments. I am ashamed to admit that my introduction to genuine cross-cultural artistic collaborations began long after my formal education: it was in Brisbane Women's Correctional Centre, where I began leading theatre projects in 2011 for my then doctoral study. Over time, more and more First Nations women from Australia and Aotearoa New Zealand joined these projects—the then General Manager suggested this was because theatre offered an outlet to explore creativity and expressiveness in ways that other prison programs did not. With these women drastically overrepresented in the system, I began offering themes and stories to explore that would be relevant to them but would nevertheless welcome non-Indigenous actors as well. I began working with Aboriginal and Torres Strait Islander artists and

> knowledge holders—people such as author and memoirist Aunty Ruth Hegarty—who, along with the women in prison, became my teachers and mentors in navigating this space. Growing up in Australia in the 1980s, I had received zero formal education about the truths of colonial domination in Australia, and through the 1990s I confess I was too distracted by partying, travelling, and working overseas. It was only once I returned to Australia and began dealing with the facts directly through the criminal justice system that I started a lifelong project of learning, guided by an exceptional group of scholars, artists, and friends. This is a work in progress.

We, Kamarra and Sarah, have been in conversation and collaboration together to varying degrees since we met at a symposium on "performance challenging stigma" in 2016 hosted by the University of Melbourne. Kamarra was there to talk about her work on *Chopped Liver*, and Sarah was presenting on *Daughters of the Floating Brothel*, one of her prison theatre projects that interrogated the legacy of female incarceration in Australia. This sparked connections, and we talked briefly about our work and agreed to stay in touch, which we did sporadically over the next few years. In February 2020, just prior to the outbreak of the COVID-19 pandemic, we reconnected in a café in Melbourne, where Sarah had just taken up a three-year research fellowship. At this meeting, Kamarra briefly outlined her ideas for shaping the next health education work—*The Score*—into a new participatory model. We both recognised an opportunity to collaborate, with Sarah's experience in applied theatre and her newfound research time and resources from the University of Melbourne, which already had links to Kamarra and Ilbijerri through the Victorian College of the Arts theatre course. With this foundation, Sarah, Kamarra, and Ilbijerri's then Social Impact Producer (Kim Bennett) and Assistant Producer (Lauren Sheree) began what would become a year of Zoom yarns about the project before we finally met in person in 2021. Through this process, we established the "looking back" part of the study (what is largely reported here) and began mapping out the development of the new model for *The Score*.

The health education works—and our investigation and reporting of them—operate at the "cultural interface" (M. Nakata 2007) between First Nations and non-Indigenous knowledges, institutions, and practices surrounding theatre, education, and wellbeing. This study therefore in part examines what it means to make work at the intersection between different cultural and political discourses, institutions, demands, and knowledges while privileging First Nations ways of knowing, being, and doing. Elsewhere, we have discussed the ethical tensions and opportunities in such work, framing our collaboration around the concept of "relational accountability" as introduced by Shawn Wilson (2008). Relationality in this case encompasses the

> Interpersonal relationships enacted within the project (among, for example team members, community participants, partners, and stakeholders), and also the 'inevitable' relationships that exist at the structural level between Indigenous and settler in social, legal and political life. (Maddison and Nakata 2020; Woodland et al. 2023, 4)

To be relationally accountable in this context means attending to all the relationships within such projects—both structural and interpersonal—in ways that are ethically and culturally grounded. As a significant part of this, we two authors are engaged in an ongoing project of "two-way mentoring and learning" (Coff and Lampert 2019), which is built on mutual respect and trust but is also able to accommodate complexity and conflict.

For the purpose of looking back, in addition to yarning together over the past several years, we consulted several primary and secondary sources to form a picture of Ilbijerri's health education works, with a particular interest in how we could learn from their successes, strengths, challenges, and tensions in moving forward with the new model. Specifically, we were interested in what the past could tell us about how we might "do" community engagement more meaningfully and how the previous works might inform how we measure "success" in the future. While these works have in some ways been framed in the past as health-focused educational performances, we aimed through this research to reframe our approach towards more holistic First Nations notions of wellbeing, which may include health outcomes directly related to programs but also encompass cultural resilience, empowerment, agency, and self-determination (see Gee et al. 2014).

Our primary research was conducted with support from Ilbijerri and approval from the University of Melbourne's Human Research Ethics Committee (ethics ID 14332). It included interviews conducted over 2020–2021 with eight practitioners who had been involved in the works over the years, which took the form of reflective yarns between Sarah,

Kamarra, and interviewees—recalling significant moments from tours, audience reception and engagement, and the strengths and challenges of the works in development, content, production, and touring. Interviewees were also asked for their input and ideas around the proposed new model. The strength of Kamarra's involvement in these yarns was that she was able to reflect more deeply on her own experience as a lead creative while also prompting memories and inviting deeper reflection from interviewees around specific moments or experiences. The practitioners interviewed had been involved in a cross section of works in a variety of roles and all agreed to be named in the research:

- Jesse Butler (Arrernte): performer in *North West of Nowhere* (2016) and *Viral* (2018–2019)
- Nazaree Dickerson (Noongar and Burmese): performer in *Chopped Liver* (2017) and community facilitator for *Scar Trees* (2019)
- Isaac Drandic (Noongar): performer in *Chopped Liver* (2006–2008)
- Shannon Hood (Kurnai and Gunditjmara) performer in *Viral* (2019)
- Mary Quinsacara (non-Indigenous): stage/tour manager for *Viral* (2018)
- Melodie Reynolds-Diarra (Wongutha-Ngadju): performer in *Chopped Liver* (2006–2008)
- Laila Thaker (Meriam Mir and Badulaig): performer in *Viral* (2018)
- Peter Waples-Crowe (Ngarigo): health worker (VACCHO and Thorne Harbour Health), member of Ilbijerri's Social Impact reference group, toured with *Body Armour*.

Sarah and Kamarra also engaged in a reflective research yarn in February 2021, from which some edited verbatim extracts are shared throughout the volume. Due to the challenges of staff turnover, organisational change, and the impacts of the COVID-19 pandemic, gaining access to thorough documentation from Ilbijerri's corporate archive for every performance was not possible; however, we were able to access the following documents and data to inform the research:

- Annual reports from 2006–2019.
- Ilbijerri's website, which contains production histories for all performances (Ilbijerri Theatre Company n.d.).

- Survey data for the *Viral* 2018 and 2019 tours and the *Scar Trees* 2019 tour. These data were gathered from audiences through the Culture Counts[5] survey platform.
- Tour debriefs, notes, and reports for the *Viral* 2018 and 2019 tours.
- Audience feedback in the hard copy guest book from the *Viral* 2018 tour and written on the set of *Viral* in 2018 and 2019.

In addition to these sources from Ilbijerri, we also consulted the evaluation report on the impact of the 2008 tour of *Chopped Liver* prepared by consulting firm Effective Change (Keating 2009) and Blayne Welsh's (2018) excellent scholarly analysis of the Hepatitis C Trilogy for the journal *Australasian Drama Studies*, written from his insider perspective as a performer in *Viral*. The data for this research were analysed using the qualitative data analysis software tool NVivo, which supports researchers in identifying key themes and patterns across different sources. These themes were then developed further through iterative research yarns and writing between we two authors.

In the next chapter, we provide a description and synopsis of each of the health education works in turn to ground the reader in the work under investigation. This is followed in Chap. 3 by a contextual review of contemporary First Nations dramaturgies in Australia, their relationship to community wellbeing, and a discussion of theatre for health education in Indigenous and global majority contexts. From Chap. 4 onwards, the book discusses each of the three most prominent themes in our data in turn. These themes are (1) the presence of **culturally led, culturally safe** practices both in creative development and performance; (2) the notion of these performances as "**gripping dramatic yarns**" that integrate strong dramaturgy and performance aesthetics with health education and messaging; and (3) the creation of **stigma-free spaces for healing, empowerment, and self-determination** through the works. These themes have been somewhat artificially separated from each other, with the acknowledgement that they normally interact in holistic ways within programs such as these. Nevertheless, by identifying them separately and exploring a range of subthemes within them, we aim to paint a holistic picture of

[5] Culture Counts is a third-party evaluation consultancy and survey platform created specifically for use by arts and culture organisations in Australia (https://culturecounts.cc/).

these works as a powerful body of culturally led, community-engaged performance practice that has much to teach us about arts-led approaches to health and wellbeing in First Nations communities and beyond.

References

Barlo, Stuart, William (Bill) Edgar Boyd, Margaret Hughes, Shawn Wilson, and Alessandro Pelizzon. 2021. Yarning as Protected Space: Relational Accountability in Research. *AlterNative: An International Journal of Indigenous Peoples* 17 (1): 40–48. https://doi.org/10.1177/1177180120986151

Bell-Wykes, Kamarra. 2018a. *Chopped Liver*. Hobart: Australian Script Centre Inc. (trading as AustralianPlays.org).

———. 2018b. *North West of Nowhere*. Hobart: Australian Script Centre Inc. (trading as AustralianPlays.org).

———. 2018c. *Body Armour*. Hobart: Australian Script Centre Inc. (trading as AustralianPlays.org).

Bessarab, Dawn, and Bridget Ng'Andu. 2010. Yarning about yarning as a legitimate method in Indigenous research. *International Journal of Critical Indigenous Studies* 3 (1): 37–50. http://hdl.handle.net/20.500.11937/37083.

Coff, Kathryn, and Jo Lampert. 2019. Mentoring as Two-Way Learning: An Australian First Nations/Non-Indigenous Collaboration. *Frontiers in Education* Vol. 4. Frontiers Media. https://doi.org/10.3389/feduc.2019.00024

Gee, Graham, Pat Dudgeon, Clinton Schultz, Amanda Hart, and Kerrie Kelly. 2014. Aboriginal and Torres Strait Islander social and emotional wellbeing. In *Working Together: Aboriginal and Torres Strait Islander Mental Health and Wellbeing Principles and Practice*, ed. Pat Dudgeon, Helen Milroy, and Roz Walker, 55–68. Canberra: Commonwealth of Australia.

Goodbye Aunty Flo. 2023. By Nazaree Dickerson. Directed by Nazaree Dickerson. Premiered at Collingwood Yards, Melbourne, Victoria, March 17.

Ilbijerri Theatre Company. n.d. We Are. Accessed August 27, 2023. https://www.ilbijerri.com.au/

Keating, Clare. 2009. *'Chopped Liver' Evaluation Report*. Effective Change Pty Ltd. Melbourne: Ilbijerri Theatre Company. Supplied.

Maddison, Sarah, and Sana Nakata. 2020. Introduction: Questioning Indigenous-settler relations. In *Questioning Indigenous-Settler Relations: Interdisciplinary Perspectives*, ed. Sarah Maddison and Sana Nakata, 1–14. Springer.

Nakata, Martin. 2007. The Cultural Interface. *The Australian Journal of Indigenous Education* 36 (S1): 7–14. https://doi.org/10.1017/S1326011100004646.

Scar Trees. 2019. By Declan Furber Gillick. Adapted by Kamarra Bell-Wykes. Directed by Kamarra Bell-Wykes. Premiered at Northcote Town Hall, Melbourne, Victoria, October 28.

Syron, Liza-Mare. 2021. *Rehearsal Practices of Indigenous Women Theatre Makers.* Springer International Publishing.

Thorner, Sabra, Fran Edmonds, Maree Clarke, and Paola Balla. 2018. Maree's Backyard: Intercultural Collaborations for Indigenous Sovereignty in Melbourne. *Oceania* 88 (3): 269–291. https://doi.org/10.1002/ocea.5206.

Viral – Are You the Cure? 2018. By Maryanne Sam. Directed by Kamarra Bell-Wykes. Various sites throughout Victoria, 2018–2019.

Welsh, Blayne. 2018. The Hepatitis C Trilogy: A Case for Indigenous Theatre as a Contemporary Manifestation of Traditional Healing Business. *Australasian Drama Studies* 73: 20–41. https://search.informit.org/doi/abs/10.3316/ielapa.146479491877297.

Wilson, Shawn. 2008. *Research is Ceremony: Indigenous Research Methods.* Fernwood.

Woodland, Sarah, Kamarra Bell-Wykes, and Carissa Lee Godwin. 2023. Yarning Up Relations: Enacting a Relational Ethics in Cross-Cultural Research-Based Theater. *Qualitative Inquiry* 29 (2): 393–402. https://doi.org/10.1177/10778004221099561.

CHAPTER 2

Ilbjierri Theatre Company: Health Education Works (2006–2019)

Abstract This chapter describes Ilbijerri Theatre Company's health education theatre productions from 2006 to 2019, led by Kamarra Bell-Wykes (co-author) in her role first as writer and later dramaturg, facilitator, and director. These works sat under Ilbijerri's Social Impact stream as separate from their mainstage productions and were funded by various state and philanthropic bodies to deliver health education and promotion around specific issues affecting Aboriginal and Torres Strait Islander communities: *Chopped Liver* (2006–2009; 2017), *Body Armour* (2010–2013) and *Viral – Are You the Cure?* (2018/2019)—also known as the Hepatitis C Trilogy—all deal with hepatitis C transmission, management, and treatment; *North West of Nowhere* (2014–2016) addresses sexual health and healthy relationships; and *Scar Trees* (2019) addresses family violence. The chapter offers an overview of the health and funding contexts in which they were created, as well as a brief snapshot of the reach and impact of each performance. We also provide a detailed synopsis of each play that includes specific approaches to writing, performance, production, and touring, before moving onto a more in-depth contextual discussion around First Nations Australian approaches to theatre in health education in Chap. 3.

Keywords First Nations theatre • Theatre in education • Applied theatre • Arts and health • Theatre for health education • Ilbijerri Theatre Company

S. Woodland, K. Bell-Wykes, *First Nations Australian Theatre for Health Equity*, https://doi.org/10.1007/978-3-031-65506-7_2

In 2005, the Victorian Department of Health first approached the nationally acclaimed Ilbijerri Theatre Company to develop a work that would address high rates of hepatitis C in First Nations communities. This became *Chopped Liver* (written by Kamarra), and since then, the health education works have been steadily evolving. The goal has been to create engaging, culturally focused ways to educate communities about pressing health and wellbeing issues; and to create spaces for open dialogue and reducing stigma around these often-sensitive topics. Since the success of *Chopped Liver*, the works have been consistently supported with funding from the Department of Health, as well as additional funding from bodies such as Creative Victoria, the Victorian Health Promotion Foundation (VicHealth), philanthropic organisations, and local government. As discussed in Chap. 1, author Kamarra Bell-Wykes, a Yuggera and Butchulla woman and successful independent theatre maker, was the driving force behind these works—first as a commissioned writer and later as a director, dramaturg, and community facilitator. Kamarra also spent five years from 2014 to 2019 in the role of Ilbijerri's Education and Learning Manager and subsequently Creative Director which enabled her to work more closely on later productions and develop her approach to community-engaged practice. Importantly for the Hepatitis C Trilogy (*Chopped Liver*, *Body Armour*, and *Viral – Are You the Cure?*), Kamarra had lived experience of having and clearing the virus, which heavily informed her creative involvement in the works. Despite their educational focus, the works have always been underpinned by an ethos of artistic excellence, with creative teams that have included some of the most recognised and esteemed Australian artists, for example, playwright and dramaturg John Romeril, performer and arts leader Rachael Maza (Ilbijerri's current Artistic Director), former Ilbijerri Artistic Director Kylie Belling, theatre makers Isaac Drandic, Margert Harvey, Declan Furber Gillick, and performers Melodie Reynolds-Diarra, Carly Sheppard, Leroy Parsons, Maurial Spearim, and Ian Michael. The works have also provided a vital platform for young and emerging First Nations artists who have gone on to work in mainstage theatre productions, film, television, education, and arts and community leadership.

The Department of Health's funding was contingent on Ilbijerri establishing a formal reference group to strategically advise on the health content of the concept, script, and production, and later community outreach for these productions. Health professionals from organisations such as the Department of Health, Victorian Aboriginal Community Controlled Health Organisation (VACCHO), and Hepatitis Victoria contributed their on-the-ground insights into their clients, target audiences, and broader health contexts, but these also inadvertently informed the characters and narratives, as will be discussed later. This ongoing structure became a vital knowledge base and created space for rigorous interrogation to ensure accurate and strength-based messaging was included that nevertheless did not impede the making of high-quality, culturally informed art.

As outlined in the Introduction, since their inception, the five health education works discussed here have reached over 26,000 audience members in tours across the country into venues ranging from traditional theatres to schools, colleges, prisons, youth justice centres, community and neighbourhood centres, health centres, housing centres, Aboriginal community-controlled organisations, university campuses, and conferences. Depending on target audiences and venues for the shows, audience members were made up of a mix of adults and young people; a mix of those directly affected by the health issues being addressed, those supporting them, and members of the wider community; and mixed gender identification. While remaining First Nations culturally focused, tours welcomed audience members from all backgrounds, with tour data from *Viral* (2018–2019) and *Scar Trees* (2019) indicating an average of 64% First Nations audience members (as compared to the national figure of 3.2% [Australian Bureau of Statistics 2022]). Tours varied in duration and reach, but typically would last approximately three weeks. The early *Chopped Liver* national tours ran up to five months and involved an average of two performances per day.

Evidence gathered over the years and for this research points towards the performances being highly successful in engaging audiences and communities with the issues through a combination of sophisticated storytelling, compelling characters, high-quality performances, humour, and cultural content. It is widely acknowledged that gathering evidence for the impact of such programs in affecting health outcomes is virtually impossible, however, the data does paint a picture of extremely high levels of audience engagement, increased insights into the issues, and evidence of audience members left feeling empowered to act in relation to their own and others' health. These findings will be explored in more depth in Chaps. 4, 5, and 6 through themes identified across all five health education works. For now, though, we discuss each of the plays in turn, beginning with the Hepatitis C Trilogy (*Chopped Liver*, *Body Armour*, and *Viral*) and followed by *North West of Nowhere* and *Scar Trees*, focusing on details about the commission, creation, production, and touring of each play. This will hopefully give the reader a strong grounding from which to understand the background and context into First Nations Australian approaches to health education through theatre (in the next chapter); and the findings and outcomes discovered through our research into these five important performances.

Chopped Liver (2006–2009 and 2017)

> She ran away.
> He ran amuck.
> And one day they ran into each other…
> Meet Lynne and Jim. They've both been around the block – working, protesting, jail, partying, and kids. Now they've come home – but can they leave their past behind?
> A Blak Comedy about life, love and being more than "chopped liver".
> *Chopped Liver* was written by Kamarra Bell-Wykes to raise awareness of hepatitis C in the Indigenous community and toured nationally from 2006 to 2009. In 2017 the show returned by popular demand and was updated to communicate that a cure is now available for hepatitis C.
> This show is deadly.[1] Hepatitis C doesn't have to be. (Ilbijerri Theatre Company n.d.-a)

Ilbijerri was commissioned in 2005 by the Victorian Department of Health to develop a play that would communicate hepatitis C prevention and education messages in a culturally appropriate way to Indigenous communities (Fig. 2.1). Ilbijerri formed a partnership with the Department of Health, the Victorian Aboriginal Community Controlled Health Organisation (VACCHO) and Hepatitis Victoria to deliver the project and contracted Kamarra Bell-Wykes as writer, John Romeril as dramaturg, and Kylie Belling as director. The artistic team worked with support from a reference group comprising the key partners, which grew in subsequent years to include Corrections Victoria, Department of Justice (who provided funding for a tour into Victorian prisons) and Justice Health (a unit of the Department of Justice). *Chopped Liver* was the work produced out of this first iteration of Ilbijerri's Social Impact stream and the first in what was to become the "Hepatitis C Trilogy" (Fig. 2.1). Arguably the most successful

[1] "Deadly" is a colloquial term for "very good" or "excellent" that is widely used by Aboriginal and Torres Strait Islander peoples in Australia.

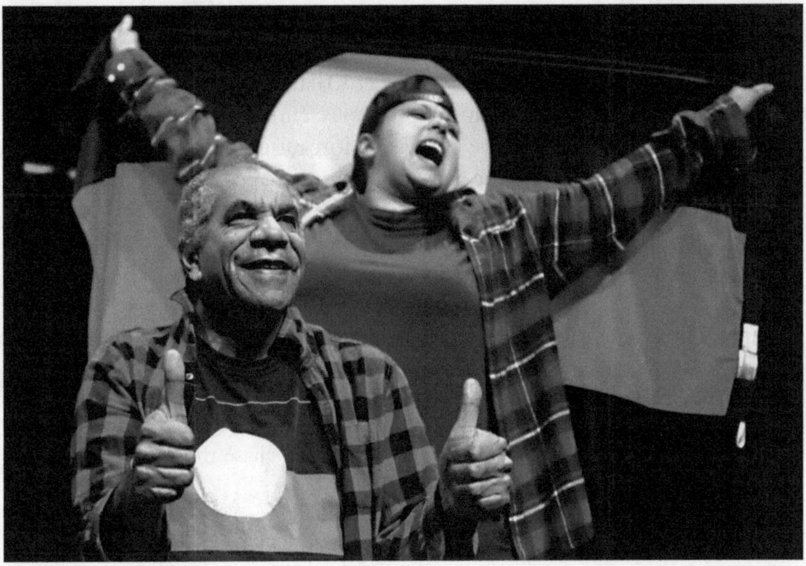

Fig. 2.1 Gregory J. Fryer (L) and Nazaree Dickerson (R), *Chopped Liver*. Image by James Henry (2017)

and well-known of the works, *Chopped Liver* provided essential creative learnings for future works. Kamarra describes the synopsis of the original play as follows:

> The play starts in 1998 and you're taken along the journey of the two characters – Lynne and Jim – over 20 years to 2006. It's about their stories. They're from a small country town – could be anywhere in Victoria. They move to Melbourne, and back again and have a kid. But the whole time that they're travelling, they're travelling with this hepatitis C virus and the play is about how their relationship with the virus changes over those 20 years. So hepatitis C is actually another character in the play. Hepatitis C is something that's from their past, in their youth. But now, 10, 15 years later, even though they've got kids, got jobs and living straight, it's something they're still living with. Mistakes they made unknowingly come back and haunt them and now it is about trying to live with their consequences. But it doesn't have to be a negative, life damaging experience. Things are what you make them, so that's what the show is trying to show. (Keating 2009, 9)

In 2017, the play returned by popular demand and was updated to include vital information about the new treatment for hepatitis C, which had much higher rates in clearing the virus than previous antiviral medications. Where the original version of the play ended with a message about how to live with the virus, the 2017 version raised awareness of the new treatment, which at that time was not being taken up by First Nations communities.

Part yarn, part stand-up comedy routine *Chopped Liver* starts with an engaging fireside-style story about a young skink who wants to be a goanna.

> Jim: There's this skink, your run of the mill, backyard skink. Not even fully grown but he's lost his tail a few times and thinks he's pretty bad. Sometimes imagines he's a mean frill-necked lizard. Then he starts thinking; maybe he's a goanna, just born in the wrong body. Do all skinks start out as skinks and the ones that chase the dream become goannas? (Bell-Wykes 2018a, 2)

Powerful imagery and cracking dialogue interweave Jim and Lynne's lives through land rights marches, the Collingwood public housing flats, and the bank of the Murray River, reflecting First Nations historical, political, and community contexts.

> Jim: 1988. Important year. The White Australian Race is having its 200th birthday. The whole world's invited to Brisbane for a big party called Expo. The Murris up there also send out an invite:
> 40, 000 years of Dreaming! 200 years of Nightmares.
> Don't Celebrate! Demonstrate! Boycott Expo 88!
> Deadly slogan hey? My cousin Johnny's catching the bus up to Brisbane. He's going to boycott Expo – And I'm going with him. Sounds to me the sort of place goannas are born! (3)

Humour and cultural metaphors "distract" the audience from the issue of the play with the first mention of hep C not coming until five minutes into the performance and working as an effective and powerful dramatic moment that packs a punch.

> Jim: The blood drips down my hands and I feel pretty tough. The ink marks my skin and I feel pretty dangerous. The virus enters my body and I don't feel a thing. Hepatitis C is so small you can't see or feel it – at first. I didn't even know I had it for another next 10 years. (10)

Inviting the audience inside hep C's lived experience transforms the characters from an infected ex-junkie and criminal to identifiable community members everyone wants to win. Repositioning hep C from an individual burden to a collective challenge creates a radical empathy in the audience that is transferrable to others and themselves.

Jim:	It was because of stigma it took us 15 years to realise hepatitis C isn't a death sentence. We, who've got living to do,
Lynne:	A kid to raise!
Jim:	I mean check us out, a good looking couple right?
SFX:	*camera click*
Lynne:	What are we: chopped liver?
Jim:	No way! (49)

With 137 performances across Melbourne, country Victoria, South Australia, New South Wales, Western Australia, Queensland, and Tasmania in 2006–2008 and 2017, *Chopped Liver* reached a total of approximately 7500 audience members touring to prisons, schools, and community organisations across the country; as well as to professional audiences at conferences and health care settings. It won the 2008 Indigenous Community Justice Award, and Victorian Public Healthcare Awards "Secretary's Award." The play set the template for Ilbijerri's cross-sectoral partnerships and artistic approach that would continue through the next 15 years and remains one of the most memorable and talked about of the Social Impact works. We will discuss some of the reasons for this further later, but in 2008, the consultancy firm Effective Change conducted an independent evaluation of the play's 2008 Victorian tour (Keating 2009). The evaluation found that the play was highly successful, largely meeting its objectives of (a) raising awareness of hepatitis C in First Nations communities; (b) developing innovative cross-sectoral partnerships to respond to the issue; (c) delivering performances in culturally appropriate community settings; (d) developing relationships between community members and health agencies; and (c) promoting and marketing the show using culturally appropriate methods and channels.

Body Armour (2011–2013)

> Meet Dannii, Harley and Rose. Three teenagers. Three individuals. Three modern-day warriors on a quest for identity; fuelled with attitude and armed with ink and steel.
> When their paths cross unexpectedly, they realise that they might have found more than they were looking for. And that sometimes, the best way to look forward is by looking back…
> *Body Armour* is the next instalment from the team behind the multi award-winning *Chopped Liver* (which has been seen by almost ten thousand people in over 150 communities, schools and prisons across Australia).
> Fresh, sassy and razor-sharp, *Body Armour* has been specifically designed for high school audiences, to raise awareness of hepatitis C in the Indigenous community and beyond.
> The story follows the journey of three teenagers as they experiment with at-risk activities such as piercing, tattooing and blood sharing. Timely comparisons to ancient body modification rituals gently remind us of the importance of history and culture in the search for identity and the need to belong.
> Vibrant, funny and non-judgemental, the show's power lies in its ability to open minds, discussions and possibilities. (Ilbijerri Theatre Company n.d.-b)

The second show in the Hepatitis C Trilogy, *Body Armour*, came from a need to target First Nations young people—who were identified as being at risk of hepatitis C—with a tailored approach that spoke specifically to their life experiences (Fig. 2.2). Employing elements of physical theatre, satire, and chorus, the work is set at the local Aboriginal community health service where the three young characters who all go to the same high school conveniently meet in the waiting room just before they are all unknowingly diagnosed with hep C. Each must overcome their individual peer pressures and support each other through what could be the most altering event of their lives. Alongside the central plot, TV archaeologist Hugh Foot investigates various traditional modification rites and their appropriation in youth culture and fashions. Body modification is presented in *Body Armour* as cultural practices integral to signifying initiation, grieving, history, kinship, and lore—drawing parallels to contemporary society and young people's search for belonging and meaning.

Hugh Foot: Meet Danielle Boye; an average Australian girl, but with a very Un-Australian body piercing. When done traditionally, a piercing was symbol of a child's rite into adulthood, perhaps the symbolism of growing older is not completely lost here in

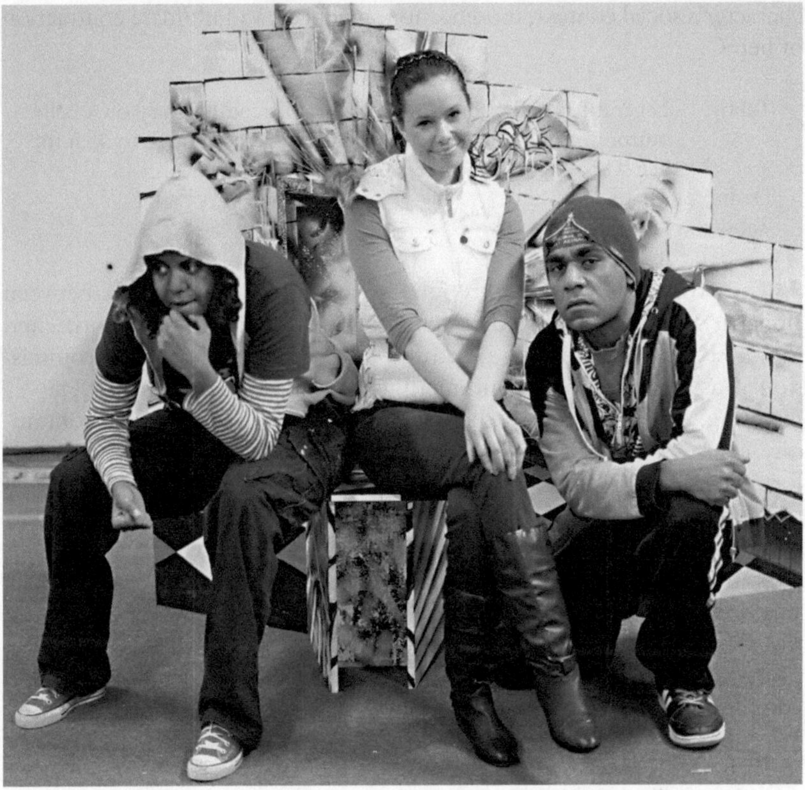

Fig. 2.2 (L-R) Maurial Spearim, Sandy Greenwood, and LeRoy Parsons, *Body Armour*. Image by James Henry (2011)

> the West or is it just another place to put pretty jewellery? Are Danni and her friends simply young women displaying their bosom buddy bond? Friendship bands merely taken to the next level? Or is this a traditional practice transformed into a modern ritual? (Bell-Wykes 2018b, 25)

Through this lens, young people are attempting to develop their own cultural frameworks of expression, belonging, identity, and experience in a modern world with modern-day risks. As their personal dynamics unfold in real-time, heightened flashbacks demonstrate the back stories of each character's social context, modification, practices, and ultimate contraction of hep C.

Tabby:	Legend has it the founding member pierced her very own belly button with it because there was no one fierce enough to do it for her. The very same needle has been used ever since.
Danni:	That's disgusting.
Tabby:	It's tradition. (16)

The work was created through the continued partnership between Ilbijerri, the Victorian Department of Health, Hepatitis Victoria, and VACCHO (whose workers joined the tour). Kamarra was again commissioned as writer, with John Romeril as dramaturg and Margaret Harvey directing. The work toured schools, justice centres, and remote community centres throughout Victoria from 2011 to 2013 and was also performed in a national regional tour across four states in 2012. In 144 performances, the show reached approximately 9600 audience members and in 2013, Ilbijerri and its project partners won the Creative Partnerships Arts and Health Award. Despite some challenges in relation to creating the work, as will be discussed later, the show was very well received. Reviewing the work in *The Age*, Cameron Woodhead described the work as a "fast paced comedy drama" and highlighted the skill of the creative team and complexity of the characters, observing:

> Each has been exposed to the virus through blood pacts, backyard tattoos, and unsterilised piercings. Far from discounting these rituals of commitment and initiation, the show suggests a rich cultural pedigree. Cod anthropology is woven into wonderfully observed clowning focused on instantly recognisable insecurities of youth—the body armour everyone wears. … Perhaps only Ilbijerri, our oldest indigenous theatre company, could speak with such empathic attunement to marginalised groups. (Woodhead 2011)

Viral – Are You the Cure? (2018–2019)

> Sifting through myths, smashing stigma, and getting the right information can seem like an impossible dream – but preventing and curing hepatitis C is now easier than you might think.

> Join Ally and Kev who live up in the flats. They've got their own little place, a brand-new baby and dreams for the future. Life should be good but sometimes things don't always go to plan.
> Meet Merv who hasn't been feeling great lately, not for some years in fact. Years of tough luck, bad choices and hard living have finally caught up with him.
> They're all looking at one final chance to make things right before it's too late. (Ilbijerri Theatre Company n.d.-e)

The third and final instalment in Ilbijerri's Hepatitis C Trilogy was *Viral*, commissioned by the Victorian Department of Health in 2018 to bring up to date the messaging and education around hep C transmission and to promote to audiences a revolutionary new, simple, and successful treatment (Fig. 2.3). Despite there now being a free, easy, safe, and effective treatment for the virus, uptake in First Nations communities was disproportionately low compared to the broader community, and the play was developed in response to this. *Viral* actor and theatre scholar Blayne Welsh (2018, 24) writes,

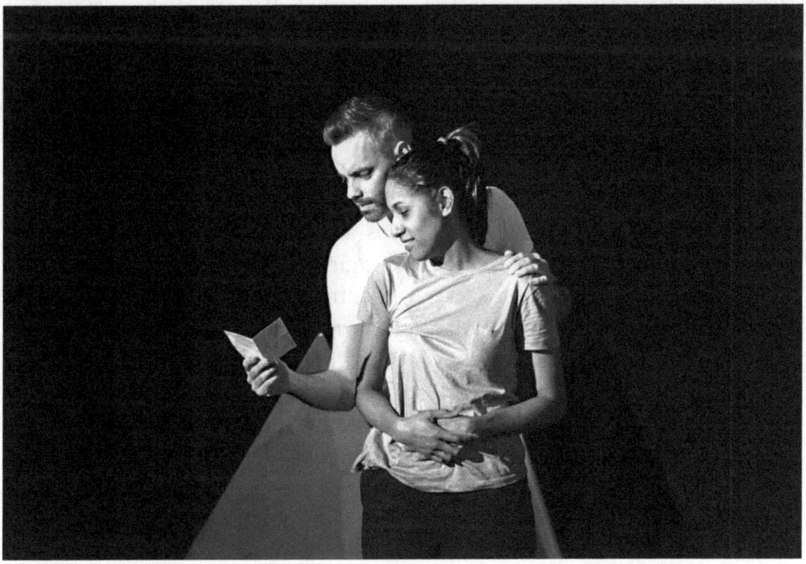

Fig. 2.3 Jesse Butler (L) and Laila Thaker (R), *Viral – Are You the Cure?* Image by Tiffany Garvie (2018)

> One of the reasons identified by the reference groups that Indigenous people living with the virus were not taking up the new treatment was due to the perceived stigmas surrounding hepatitis C, including its association with drug use and the fear of being shamed by community and family should their status become public.

As with the previous two works, a key goal was to explore the unique complexities of hep C in the First Nations context and break down the shame and stigma associated with the virus through live performance and comedy. Kamarra was again brought on board as a lead creative, this time in the role of director, dramaturg, and community facilitator, with multi-arts practitioner and Ilbijerri founding member Maryanne Sam commissioned to write the script.

From 2014 to 2019, Kamarra was appointed in an ongoing role at Ilbijerri and began exploring ways to embed more community-engaged approaches in developing the Social Impact works. This led to community workshops and yarning circles becoming integral to the theme and story development for *Viral* and *Scar Trees* (see further below) and formed the basis for the approach being trialled through the new model underpinning *The Score*. The strengths, opportunities, and challenges of these strategies will be explored later; however, Kamarra's desire to engage with First Nations communities directly for *Viral* was borne out of a need to answer the fundamental question of why people were not taking up treatment. Having cleared the virus over six years earlier under the old treatment regime, Kamarra did not feel confident in understanding the barriers that faced communities in 2018. For this reason, she worked with Shiralee Hood to design and facilitate workshops with three groups who were seen as being important targets for the messaging. These were active IV drug users who were either not seeking the treatment or were in the pre-contemplation or contemplation stage in relation to treatment; incarcerated adults who may or may not have had the opportunity to take up the treatment; and older women in regional areas who were considering, undergoing, or completing the treatment. These workshops greatly informed the characters and underlying themes, including shame and self-worth, intergenerational relationships and trauma, communal sharing practices,[2] and daily survival, distrust of the colonial health system and its medicines, and historical and ongoing systemic failure. As a result of *Chopped Liver*'s previous success and the status and expertise of Kamarra and Shiralee as facilitators, these workshops also resulted in strong community buy-in for the work.

For *Viral* Kamarra, as director, developed various scenes, themes, and characters with the actors and playwright using improvising and devising techniques drawn from the community workshops, fictionalising the dramatic elements, and developing the creative team's understanding about the issue. The playwright (Maryanne Sam) then developed these ideas into the script and the process was repeated back and forth to reach the final draft. Informed by the community workshops, the team developed three characters at different stages of the virus: Ally and Doc/Kev—a young couple with a newborn baby—and Merv, Ally's estranged father. Ally contracted hep C from Doc sharing needles but is now clean and considering the treatment. Doc is still using, in and out of jail, and doesn't see the point. Merv, who has contracted hep C through a transplant and has recently been hospitalised for liver failure, reaches out to Ally hoping to meet his grandson before he dies.

Doc: How long have I had it?
Used for about 12 years. So, ten I guess.
Ally: A couple of years
Merv: Too long.
How did I get It?
They give it to me. Kidney transplant. Had a blood transfusion
Ally: Can I pass?
Doc: The usual. Treatment?
Nah! I can get rid of it meself mate.
Merv: They're not getting their hands on me again. Not after what they done.

Viral centralises Ally's perspective who must decide to choose the treatment with or without her partner, a common challenge faced by women

[2] Communal sharing practices refers to community/family practices of sharing food/possessions and naturally extends to sharing needles amongst family members participating in an intravenous lifestyle.

who often prioritise others over their own needs. These intersecting narratives reflect the testimonies and complexities of the communities' experiences.

Merv: Few aches and pains. They can't keep me down.
Doc: Comin down's worse! Dying? Dyin's easy. It's livin that's hard.
Merv: I'm not going anywhere! Got my girl Maggie out there somewhere.
Ally: Thinking about it a lot lately. I don't want my son growing up without his Mum. Not like I did.

Alongside the central plotline, a problematic production crew is filming the characters' lives for a budget documentary about hep C. These modern White archetypes add humour and a satirical lens that interrogates the health care system and society's stereotypes and misconceptions about hep C and First Nations communities while being an efficient vehicle to distribute health information.

Lewis: We've got a broad selection of Koooorees from the community lined up; Elders, young couples, prisoners, those in different stages of treatment and those who don't seek help at all.
Lizzie: I'm so excited. Let's close this gap.
Phil: I don't get it. Why don't they get the treatment?
Liz: Coz they've got their bush medicines and stuff
Phil: But this actually works and it's free.
Lewis: Well, as the doco title alludes to Phillip, 'Viral – Are You the Cure?' That is exactly what we're about to find out!

Viral had the most sophisticated design of all the works, elevating the production both aesthetically and dramatically. Rather than basic song samples and sound effects as used in previous productions, multi-instrumentalist and sound designer "small sound" composed an original symphonic score. The music provided the intensity and creative quality of a "professional" mainstage production while supporting the audience's emotional connection to the piece. Also designed and constructed by small sound, the set—coined "The Viragon"—consisted of six large triangles and a central circular piece that interlocked to create a raised hexagon platform (and subsequently replicating the DNA shape/structure of hep C). Originally designed as a portable stage to overcome the limited eyelines of non-theatre venues, it instead creatively informed the work in a much deeper way, its fragmented pieces forming the play's various institutional settings housing commission flats, prisons, and the hospital. As the characters reunited with their inner strength, the Viragon was finally arranged in its complete form and danced upon in celebration (the only time it was used as a stage), symbolising their victory over the virus. After the show, audiences were encouraged to sign and leave comments on the Viragon creating a communal message board crossing regions and prison walls, this transference of energy and purpose transformed a set into a political act and a performance into a ceremony.

Ultimately, every theatrical element of *Viral* including the set, soundtrack, and even scene transitions were informed by the social and cultural context of the virus and its lived experience. This conscious and instinctual exchange between the issue, the community, and the art created the most sophisticated creative product and engaged audiences for the works thus far. *Viral* toured to community centres, schools, and prisons across Victoria and South Australia in 2018 and throughout Victoria in 2019 delivering 34 performances to around 2061 audience members. The planned 2020 tour was cancelled due to the COVID-19 pandemic, which led Ilbijerri to develop the play into a digital film and educational resource that was launched in July 2022 (Ilbijerri n.d.-e), which, despite having the same characters and plot lines, was ultimately a much more sombre and potentially less engaging work.

North West of Nowhere (2014–2016)

> One ute, two teenagers and a long road ahead. No looking back now.
>
> Wyatt and Nella are 16 and from the middle of nowhere. Wyatt's in love with a girl who doesn't love him back and Nella just wants to escape from the small town gossip. Enter Cuz. He's just got out of jail and knows a good time when he sees one. Desperate to fit in, Wyatt tags along with Nella and Cuz and together they pile into Cuz's ute headed one way for Sydney. Nella's got her heart set on the big smoke and a whole new life, Cuz has other ideas and Wyatt can't help thinking they should all just turn back now.
>
> *North West of Nowhere* is the next instalment from the team behind the multi award-winning shows *Chopped Liver* and *Body Armour*, which have been seen by almost 20,000 people in over 200 communities, schools and prisons across Australia.
>
> *North West of Nowhere* is raw, honest and takes a fresh approach to raising awareness of sexual health and the importance of respectful sexual relationships.

> Written specifically for secondary school audiences, young people will relate to Wyatt and Nella as they journey from their teenage dreams to proud young adults ready for the world. (Ilbijerri Theatre Company n.d.-c)

North West of Nowhere is the first of two performances under discussion that sits outside the Hepatitis C Trilogy (Fig. 2.4). The play was developed again in partnership with Victoria's Department of Health in response to a spike in rates of chlamydia and other sexually transmissible infections (STIs) among First Nations young people, exacerbated by high-risk sexual behaviours and attitudes. Building on their previous work on *Chopped Liver* and *Body Armour*, Ilbijerri again commissioned Kamarra Bell-Wykes as writer and John Romeril as dramaturg, with input from the reference group. Rachael Maza directed the 2014–2015 iterations of the show, with Eva Grace Mullaley directing a remount in 2016.

The play was created for secondary school-aged audiences and followed what Kamarra describes as a standard Theatre in Education (TIE) format, with the performance followed by a facilitated audience discussion. As with

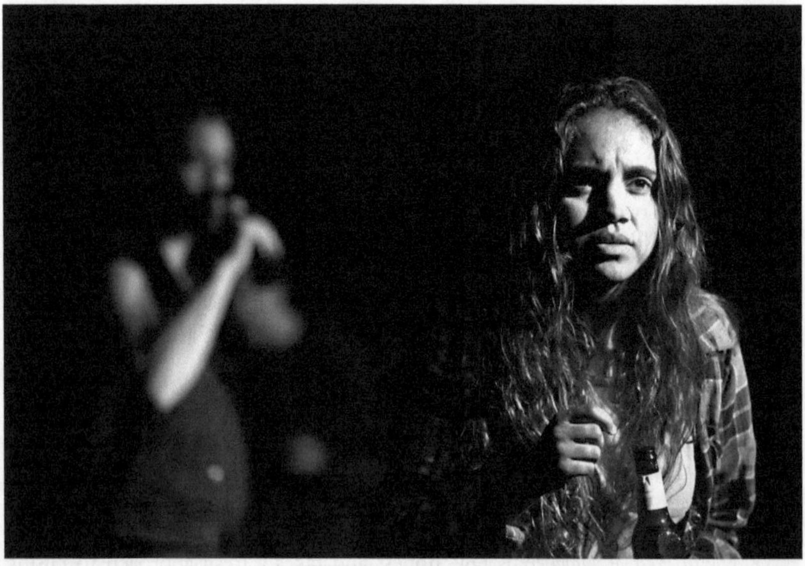

Fig. 2.4 Jesse Butler (L) and Brandi Nelson (R), *North West of Nowhere*. Image by James Henry (2016)

the other productions, Kamarra focused on the wider social context informing the central message. It was about negotiating respectful sexual relationships and about young people coming into their power to be able to ask for the respect and make choices that honour themselves—particularly within a sexual health space. The characters, therefore, needed to journey from a place of disempowerment and self-comprise to one of power and pride.

Set on Survival Day Eve,[3] *North West of Nowhere* is a coming-of-age road-trip story focused on 16-year-old best friends Nella and Wyatt, who ultimately journey from disempowerment to self-determination and pride. The two older male characters offer opposing male role models for the two young protagonists. Ol' Man is an engaging narrator appearing as a mysterious shapeshifter along the journey, guiding and aiding the young travellers on their way. In opposition to Ol' Man (played by the same actor) is Wyatt's Cuz (cousin), a charming bad boy who comes with big risks and even bigger consequences whilst bringing humour and energy to the piece.

> Wyatt: Looks just like Dad, pumped up and inked out from the last stint inside.
> Nella: Kinda bloke just looks at a woman and breaks her heart.
> Wyatt: Checking out the barmaid, checking out anything with a pulse.
> Nella: A man's man, a real lady killer. Kinda bloke looks at a woman and her clothes just fall off.
> Wyatt: Kinda son my Dad wanted – kinda man I'll never be. (Bell-Wykes 2018c, 8)

Each of the protagonists' character arc in *North West of Nowhere* is underpinned by cultural metaphors, grounding their journey in ancestral wisdom and experience. Wyatt's arc is paralleled by a fictionalised retelling of the Bogong Moth's Song-line from Queensland to Capital Territory, a tale of strength and transformation Wyatt must replicate.

> Ol' Man: Just when he thinks he can't fly any further he lands on the mountains peak, stretches his wings and dances in the water. Can you hear the mountain calling you little fulla? It's telling you – it's time, you're ready for change. (25)

[3] "Survival Day" (also called "Invasion Day") is a replacement name given to Australia Day (26 January), on which settler society marks the arrival in 1788 of the First Fleet of convict ships from Britain.

Nella's metaphor is drawn from The Dreaming story of the Brolga Dancer, a beautiful young woman held captive by a Magic Man who forbids her from dancing, reflecting Nella's experience with her abusive boyfriend.

Ol' Man:	But when she stretched her wings she found she still could, it could not be stolen; her spirit was stronger than any man's magic. (44)

As Nella and Wyatt overcome their internal and external battles, they must overcome various external challenges that ultimately lead them to Canberra and the historically significant 40th anniversary of the Tent Embassy,[4] reclaim their determination and purpose as young Blackfullas with their whole future in front of them.

Nella:	Feel it in my bones.
Wyatt:	Rhythm in my feet.
Nella:	Rises in my chest.
Wyatt:	Song lines like a heartbeat.
Nella and Wyatt:	I wasn't ready for this.
Nella:	I can't.
Wyatt:	I'm right here by your side.
Nella:	Stand on the circles edge.
Wyatt:	Red cloth of lap laps, white ochre on brown skin.
Nella:	Bare feet stomp and sweep Imprint the black ground underneath.
Wyatt:	They all turn to look.
Nella:	Like they've been waiting.
Nella and Wyatt:	For us to come. (43–44)

The show toured schools and communities across Victoria in 2014, 2015, and 2016, reaching around 7112 audience members through 83 performances. It was also shared in several important health sector contexts, including the International HIV/AIDS Conference (2014), the

[4] The Aboriginal Tent Embassy was originally established in 1972 by a group of activists who set up in front of Parliament House to protest oppressive government policies. It was permanently established on the lawns of Parliament House in 1992 and remains as a site of protest for Aboriginal and Torres Strait Islander peoples seeking sovereignty and self-determination (National Museum of Australia 2022).

Department of Health (2015), and the Centre for Excellence in Rural Sexual Health's (CERSH) SexRurality Conference (2015). *North West of Nowhere* was also unique in that the 2015 tour was supported by a First Nations health worker who facilitated the post-show discussions and worked to connect young people with relevant local health services; and a web-based educational resource accompanying the performance was produced by Ilbijerri's Marguk education program.

Scar Trees (2019)

> Kirra-Lee and Bryce are at the servo. The jerry can is half-full. One phone's flat and the other one's out of credit.
> Garren's on his BMX. The shit one. He knows all about what it can do, and its limits. He knows the tracks he doesn't want to go down. Fightin an that. He knows there's other ways. There's gotta be other ways.
> Uncle Laurie does his wood carving and runs a men's group. He's been off the grog for a while now.
> They're all trying to get to Uncle Pat's funeral. But when they get there, what stories will be told, and what will be left unspoken? (Ilbijerri Theatre Company n.d.-d)

The last of the health education plays discussed in this volume is *Scar Trees*, created in 2019 with funding from Creative Victoria and the Victorian Health Promotion Foundation (VicHealth) and aimed to address family violence in First Nations communities (Fig. 2.5). Part of the approach was to implement community workshops with children and young people in care to explore the issue of family violence from their perspective and develop a script from these. For support with this element of the project, they approached the Victorian Aboriginal and Child Care Agency (VACCA). Arrernte playwright Declan Furber Gillick was commissioned to write the original script, but due to time and geographical constraints on the collaborative process, Kamarra (in her capacity as director and dramaturg) adapted the script in rehearsals.

Scar Trees is a naturalistic character-driven drama that offers a powerful reflection of the emotional truths of family violence. Focused on 15-year-old Garren, in and out of care, he demonstrates the lived reality of crisis experienced by young people trapped in cycles of generational dysfunction, systematic failings, and violence. Established via a troubled and compelling

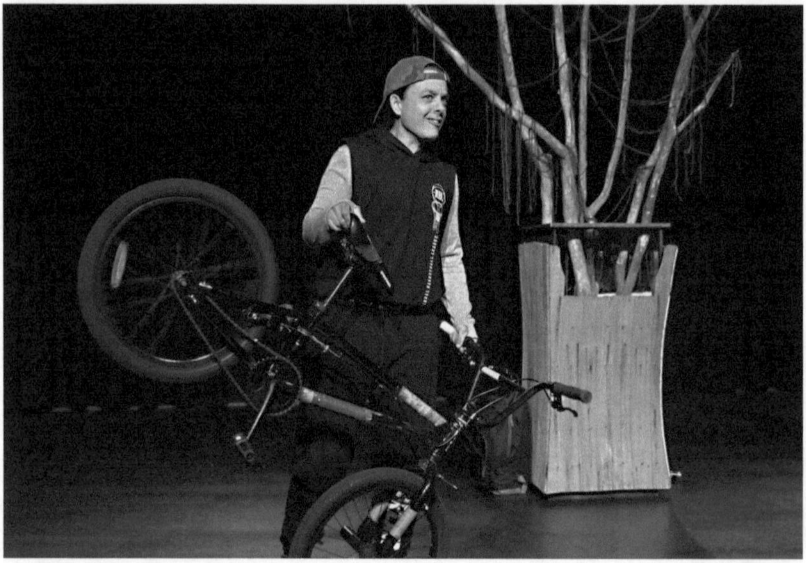

Fig. 2.5 Racheal Oak Butler, *Scar Trees.* Image by Tiffany Garvie (2019)

monologue whilst popping wheelies on his BMX bike, the audience is playfully drawn into the young man's abandonment and trauma.

Garren: Yeah, nah, this one's gammon.[5] My dad got me a proper BMX. A Haro CK AM. Yeah, he got me it. But it's at his house. In Ascot Vale. Yeah, I had to leave my bike at dad's. I had to leave dad's cos one of the kids - my foster brother or step brother or whatever - he said my mum was a prostitute. And I was like – she's not and who cares if she is but she's not. But he said some other shit. Full dirty shit. I won't tell you what he said but yeah anyway, I went in that place what I go into when it's… All I can hear is like 'roooaaarrrw' like in my ears. All I can hear is like roaring like I'm standing on the ring road with all the cars plus a plane is going over. Like that's all I can hear. And all I can see is white.

[5] 'Gammon' is a colloquial term used in many Aboriginal and Torres Strait Islander communities to refer to being fake, inauthentic, cheap, or broken.

Garren's carer, Uncle Laurie, offers a flawed and engaging role model that demonstrates the impacts of colonisation and intergenerational trauma redeemed through unconditional love, self-compassion, and personal healing.

Uncle Laurie: I started to do me carvin'. I went down the back and got my tools and they was still sharp. Hadn't got rusty or nothin'. Sharp as I'd left 'em wrapped up in the cloth in their spot above the generator. And I never touched a drop since. Can ask your Aunty Dot, any of me grannies, anyone like that. Anyone who's been around me these last eight years. I'll guarantee you there's no-one alive or dead that'd tell you they preferred me on the grog.

The second plot line follows siblings, 18-year-old Kirra-Lee and 22-year-old Bryce, broken down at a regional petrol station on their way to their father's funeral. Kirra, obsessed with photography, carries a camera everywhere as she documents the world around her, the good, the bad, and the ugly.

Kirra-Lee points the camera at Bryce

Bryce: Kirra! I'm eatin' a pie!
Kirra: Yup
Bryce: What you gotta point that at me for?
Kirra: This is the real shit, Bryce
Bryce: Whatchu mean 'the real shit'? No one wanna see a black bastard eatin' a pie!

Their playful and sometimes explosive relationship portrays a familiar family dynamic full of humour and tension. As they reflect on their father's death, Bryce and Kirra's opposing views of his domestic abuse collide and its impacts on their lives emerge.

Kirra: Well you'll get your chance to say your bit, then, won't you? You'll get your chance to say your bit. Cos every bastard and his dog wants to hear your bit. Cos everyone's a hero when they're dead.
Bryce: We're gonna feel it differently. We're gonna have different feelings about it. And different memories. You got yours. And I got mine. And I got a right to remember the father I remember.

The intersecting narratives offer the victims, observers, and perpetrators differing perspectives on violence, exploring a multi-layered portrayal of its causes and transgenerational impacts.

Bryce: Who would stay in a situation like that? You probably don't remember. You probably remember it worse than it was cos you were scared.

Kirra: You don't just leave, Bryce. You can't just…leave. I thought you were smarter than that. Really, honestly I did. You live in a little bubble, ay. You live in a little bubble of thinking the world is all good. That our father was a good man who loved the footy, loved his family, done so much for his people. And used to have a bit too much 'sometimes' and pushed mum around 'once or twice'.

Building on the elevated design of *Viral*, *Scar Trees* also featured an original musical score and metaphorical set design with a large makeshift scar tree doubling as a petrol bowser set centre stage. The tree's large and almost mythical presence divided the space in two to create a split-screen device of two separate worlds of Garren and Uncle Laurie and the stranded siblings. A mesmerising dance of power dynamics and tension unfolds between the characters as the narratives cross back and forth before finally colliding in an explosive climax where the extent of the abuse and the family and community's complicity is revealed in a confrontational but accurate demonstration of the perpetration, enabling and protecting of family violence.

Garren: People say you can't say nothin'. It's just our way. Private. What happens behind closed doors…gotta stay there. Well, if that's true, I'm never goin' behind a closed door. I'll keep my door open, thank you very much. Cos there's other ways. There's gotta be other ways. Not like in the movies. Not happily ever after. Not Disney shit. Just like, takin' care. Takin' care of each other. Cos you want to. Cos you can. Cos, like, maybe even you're good at it. Cos you know how, that's all. And cos it's the right thing to do.

Through the community workshops, the work aimed to empower the young people and engage community audiences with a focus on the experiences of victim-survivors of domestic and family violence. Some tensions within this approach are explored further later, however, the work was premiered at Melbourne's Northcote Town Hall then toured throughout Victoria into health and community centres in 17 performances to a total of around 703 audience members. Again, this work included in the tour personnel the role of Family Violence Support Coordinator—a facilitator role that was responsible for "facilitate[ing] the yarning circles after each performance and to set it up as a safe space for community to give feedback after watching the show, but also unpack anything that may have come up as a result of watching the show" (Nazaree Dickerson, interview, 2021).

Conclusion

For the creation of the five works described above, a 'traditional Western' creative process was utilised involving 18-month writing periods and ongoing dramaturgical and creative development support with varying degrees of community and artistic success, often depending on the ability to balance each of these components in ways that would yield the best possible result. Despite some of the tensions in trying to achieve this balance, a growing list of best-practice principles and creative processes for delivering socially responsive, culturally informed, high-quality art while maximising community impact has emerged.

- Get to the heart of it: What's the play about? What's the play *really* about? For example, *Chopped Liver* is a play about hep C, but it is *really* about shame, love, and redemption.
- Systemic issues and the human condition: What are the social and spiritual factors underlying the high-risk behaviours? What are the deeper beliefs and societal systems that inform and underpin high-risk behaviours such as sharing needles, having unprotected sex, or not getting tested?
- A meaningful narrative of achievable transformation: Identify the problem, its underlying causes and opportunities for internal and external transformation through the characters and narratives to achieve pathways out of the "problem."
- We don't make pamphlets we make theatre: Our job isn't to teach facts but to evoke feelings and create a space for honest, compassionate discussion about stigmatised issues.
- A spoon full of sugar helps the medicine go down: 98% creativity, 2% health information.

- Get 'em laughing then punch 'em in the guts! Win your audience over with humour then floor them with emotion.
- Our stories told our way by us: Authentic representation of First Nations languages, culture, knowledges, histories, social issues, and contexts is essential to creating empowering transformative work and audience buy-in.
- Western problems need cultural solutions: Colonial challenges take cultural resilience to survive.
- Identifiable, marginalised, but redeemable characters who offer the broadest representation of the issue and serve as the strongest vehicles for both the narrative and the health information.
- High-quality work that meets the target audiences' needs and creative aesthetic, i.e. a play for young people needs a different approach from one created for Elders.
- Safe and dangerous: The work must safely and truthfully represent the issue and the relevant high-risk behaviours and contributing factors.
- No magic solutions: Brutal honesty and realistic optimism that accurately represents the lived reality of the target audience.
- Act local, think local—processes, narrative, characters, themes, language, and most importantly, cultural material should be drawn from and reflected back to the people it is intended for, i.e. the fiction should reflect and respect the beliefs and systems of the context the performance is being created for.

We return to these critical factors in more detail throughout the study, however, this summary list is intended to provide the reader with a strong grounding in how Kamarra and Ilbijerri approach the creation of such works. The next chapter offers a review of contemporary First Nations dramaturgies in Australia and a discussion of theatre for health education in First Nations and global majority contexts. This will demonstrate how the five works discussed here are situated within a strong legacy of contemporary First Nations theatre making in Australia that centres dramaturgies of community wellbeing, strength, and resistance.

References

Australian Bureau of Statistics. 2022. Census of Population and Housing - Counts of Aboriginal and Torres Strait Islander Australians. Accessed August 14, 2023. https://www.abs.gov.au/statistics/people/aboriginal-and-torres-strait-islander-peoples/census-population-and-housing-counts-aboriginal-and-torres-strait-islander-australians/2021

Bell-Wykes, Kamarra. 2018a. *Chopped Liver*. Canberra: Australian Script Centre Inc. (trading as AustralianPlays.org).

———. 2018b. *Body Armour*. Canberra: Australian Script Centre Inc. (trading as AustralianPlays.org).

———. 2018c. *North West of Nowhere*. Canberra: Australian Script Centre Inc. (trading as AustralianPlays.org).

Ilbijerri Theatre Company. n.d.-a. *Body Armour*: Victorian Tour. Accessed August 14, 2023. https://www.ilbijerri.com.au/event/body-armour/

———. n.d.-b. *Chopped Liver*: Victorian Tour. Accessed August 14, 2023. https://www.ilbijerri.com.au/event/chopped-liver/

———. n.d.-c. *North West of Nowhere*: Touring Victoria. Accessed August 14, 2023. https://www.ilbijerri.com.au/event/northwest-of-nowhere/

———. n.d.-d. *Scar Trees*: Adapted from the Original Script by Declan Furber Gillick. Accessed August 14, 2023. https://www.ilbijerri.com.au/event/scar-trees/

———. n.d.-e. *Viral*: Watch Now. Accessed August 14, 2023. https://www.ilbijerri.com.au/event/viral-film/

Keating, Clare. 2009. *'Chopped Liver' Evaluation Report*. Effective Change Pty Ltd. Melbourne: Ilbijerri Theatre Company. Supplied.

National Museum of Australia. 2022. Defining Moments: Aboriginal Tent Embassy. Accessed August 25, 2023. https://www.nma.gov.au/defining-moments/resources/aboriginal-tent-embassy

Scar Trees. 2019. By Declan Furber Gillick. Adapted by Kamarra Bell-Wykes. Directed by Kamarra Bell-Wykes. Premiered at Northcote Town Hall, Melbourne, Victoria, October 28, 2019.

Viral – Are You the Cure?. 2018. By Maryanne Sam. Directed by Kamarra Bell-Wykes. Various sites throughout Victoria, 2018–2019.

Welsh, Blayne. 2018. The Hepatitis C Trilogy: A Case for Indigenous Theatre as a Contemporary Manifestation of Traditional Healing Business. *Australasian Drama Studies* 73: 20–41. https://search.informit.org/doi/abs/10.3316/ielapa.146479491877297.

Woodhead, Cameron. 2011. Body Armour. *The Age*, July 22 2011. https://www.theage.com.au/entertainment/theatre/body-armour-20110721-1hqqs.html-https://www.theage.com.au/entertainment/theatre/body-armour-20110721-1hqqs.html.

CHAPTER 3

Theatre in Health and Wellbeing: A First Nations Australian Approach

Abstract The health education theatre works produced by Ilbijerri Theatre Company since 2006 represent a contemporary continuation of cultural storytelling, performance, education, and healing ceremonies that have been practised by Australian First Nations communities for millennia. While these works can be seen as standalone examples of First Nations theatre practice, they also intersect with theatre in education, theatre in health education, and theatre for development—collectively situated under the banner of 'applied theatre' in Western theatre studies. The integration of contemporary Australian First Nations performance practice with applied theatre is unique, making a study of these works significant for a global audience. This chapter provides a contextual review of contemporary First Nations dramaturgies in Australia and their relationship to community wellbeing, strength, and resistance. It is followed by a discussion of focused theatre for health education programs in First Nations and global majority contexts. By bringing together these strands, we aim to situate the health education works produced by Ilbijerri within a theoretical framework that extends beyond the notion of 'social impact' into a more holistic conception of wellbeing that offers a foundation for subsequent discussion in the book.

Keywords First Nations theatre • Theatre in education • Applied theatre • Arts and health • Theatre for health education

S. Woodland, K. Bell-Wykes, *First Nations Australian Theatre for Health Equity*, https://doi.org/10.1007/978-3-031-65506-7_3

The performance works examined in this volume represent a contemporary continuation of cultural storytelling, performance, education, and healing ceremony that have been practised by Australian First Nations communities for millennia (Welsh 2018). It is beyond our scope to undertake a full review of scholarly research on such performance practices, but this remains a critical underpinning for the works under examination, and we return to these ideas throughout the study. Viewed through the lens of Western theatre studies, the works can be seen as stand-alone examples of contemporary First Nations theatre practice but also as sitting within areas that have been variously described as theatre in education (TIE), theatre in health education (THE), and theatre for development (TfD)—all forms that are often collected under the broader banner of applied theatre (Prendergast and Saxton 2016). This branch of theatre studies recognises the inherent qualities of theatre—its capacity to aesthetically engage people through a live, communal, immediate event—as a powerful portal to transformative social change (whether educational, political, cultural, or therapeutic). The integration of contemporary Australian First Nations performance practice with contemporary applied theatre is unique, which we suggest makes a study of these works significant for a global audience. This chapter therefore consists of a broad contextual review encompassing contemporary First Nations dramaturgies in Australia and their relationship to community wellbeing, followed by a review of theatre for health education in First Nations and global majority contexts. By bringing together these strands, the chapter aims to situate Ilbijerri's health education performances within a theoretical framework that extends beyond the notion of social impact to offer a foundation for subsequent discussions in the book.

First Nations Theatre in Australia: Dramaturgies of Wellbeing, Strength, and Resistance

Since their inception, Kamarra has been employed as a lead creative in most of the health education works produced by Ilbijerri (aside from the most recent production, *Goodbye Aunty Flo,* which was written and directed by Nazaree Dickerson). Outside of these projects, Kamarra has also worked in strong artistic collaborations, creating independent productions such as *Chase* (2022), *Whose Gonna Love 'Em? I am that I AM* (2022), and *A Nightime Travesty* (2023). Her performance collective A

Night Daylight Connection[1] brings a unique vision to the contemporary theatre landscape, producing challenging, visceral, darkly funny works that disrupt the limiting narratives and expectations often associated with First Nations Australian theatre on the mainstage (Nair et al. 2023). Kamarra brings this sensibility to the health education works, arguing that they must be well crafted, energetic, and engaging to deliver their educational goals successfully. Ilbijerri Theatre Company itself boasts a three-decade history of producing highly successful First Nations Australian stories for the stage, with many of their plays achieving international success and critical acclaim, and becoming established in the canon of Australian theatre (Casey 2013).

This body of work sits within a broader context of contemporary First Nations theatre making in Australia that first gained prominence in the 1960s and 1970s, which was led in part by the production of Kevin Gilbert's 1968 play *The Cherry Pickers* (Gilbert 1988) and the establishment of the National Black Theatre in 1972. The works produced combined traditional Aboriginal or Torres Strait Islander performance traditions with Anglo-European theatre conventions and were seen to bring unique "innovations of form" to the Australian stage (Casey and Craigie 2011), building on a continuous legacy of contributions to Western theatre since the first European settlements (Casey 2000, 86). It is beyond our scope to examine this history in detail, but these works are seen as processes of continuous storytelling, adaptation, and survival over millennia—in the contemporary settler context, contributing to assertions of sovereignty and representation, achieving reconciliation and truth telling, and providing spaces to heal from the traumas of colonisation (Bracknell et al. 2021; Casey 2000; Enoch 2002; Perkins 2000; Syron 2021).

Contemporary Australian First Nations dramaturgies are invariably situated at the "interface" (Nakata 2007) with non-Indigenous (or Western) performance traditions—one that is often troubled by questions of ownership, representation, and the oppressive legacies of colonisation (Lo and Gilbert 2002; Syron 2021). Acclaimed Aboriginal playwright and arts leader Wesley Enoch (2002, 14) highlighted the interdisciplinarity of First

[1] A Daylight Connection comprises Kamarra Bell-Wykes, Carly Sheppard, and smallsound plus guest artists. They are a resident company at Malthouse Theatre in Melbourne Victoria (2023) producing, in their words, a "unique brand of post-traumatic adventure theatre" (Malthouse Theatre 2023).

Nations performance as being "commonplace," with the integration of art forms such as painting, dance, and song: "The 'theatre' or ritual and play is made of ... relationships between artforms." Susan Thurow (2018, 132–133) observes that the "particular cultural horizon" of contemporary First Nations theatre remains grounded through these interdisciplinary practices. Syron (2021, 108–109) suggests that trying to define "Indigenous theatre" as a discrete genre is therefore unhelpful, instead examining "what makes a work Indigenous?" She goes on to explore how Indigenous sovereignty and ownership are asserted through performance development and rehearsal practices. This accords strongly with Kamarra and other contemporary performance makers who seek to decolonise rehearsal and performance spaces by centring First Nations cultures and practices (Bracknell et al. 2021; Hyland et al. 2018; Neumeier 2014) and challenging the dominance of non-Indigenous producers and arts leaders who stage works in ways that perpetuate colonial power relations (Boehme 2018). This is relevant to the health education works under examination here, with added complexities such as how Anglo-centric frameworks for health and wellbeing interact with the creation of these works. We now introduce some further elements within contemporary Australian First Nations dramaturgy that are of critical importance in examining the health education works.

Establishing deep and ethical community collaborations and reciprocal relations, both within and beyond the rehearsal space, is a critical feature of most First Nations-led theatre practices. This reflects the strong sense of obligation to family, community, and Country among Aboriginal and Torres Strait Islander artists (Thorner et al. 2018) and a recognition that knowledge that is generated and transmitted through performance is a shared project that requires adherence to cultural protocols (Harvey 2018). This can include consulting with Elders and knowledge holders to ensure that cultural processes and representations within works are respectfully and appropriately conducted (Bracknell et al. 2021). Citing Ilbijerri Artistic Director Rachael Maza (2015), Liza-Mare Syron (2021, 3–4) suggests that "ownership" in Indigenous theatre encompasses both the individual ownership of creatives and the collective ownership of communities. We have previously drawn on Opaskwayak Cree scholar Shawn Wilson's (2008) theorising of relationality as integral to Indigenous ontologies and epistemologies, which encompasses relations with people, with the environment/land, with the cosmos, and with ideas. For Wilson (2008), ethics in Indigenous research involves "relational accountability," which forms a key aspect of Kamarra's approach to performance making and our thinking around the health education works (Woodland et al. 2023). Relational accountability can be seen to inform how First Nations stories are represented on the stage, as discussed further below, as well as how cultural safety[2] is maintained in the process of making and presenting works (see also Bracknell et al. 2021). In a contemporary settler context, this approach contributes to the decolonising project, removing the hierarchical (colonial) structures of Anglo-European rehearsal and performance spaces.

Kathryn Kelly and Emily Coleman (2019, 53) discuss how "community engagement" has become prevalent in the Australian performing arts landscape, with artists and companies promising (sometimes uncritically) that works will provide "connection, collective endeavour and reciprocity without expectation." However, in the context of Aboriginal and Torres Strait Islander performance practice, this carries a much deeper resonance that infuses all aspects of the work. Ilbijerri has always naturally integrated community engagement with their mainstage theatre work, an approach that Kelly and Coleman (2019, 56) argue shifts the binaries between "community" and "professional" arts practice, which in their view contributes to "showing the important contribution of Aboriginal knowledge frameworks to the Australian performance sector." Nevertheless, to speak to mainstream narratives of arts policy and practice in Australia, Ilbijerri has categorised the health education works discussed here as part of their "Social Impact Program" (Ilbijerri Theatre Company n.d.), separating them from their mainstage works. However, First Nations efforts towards health, education, and activism are most frequently intertwined with artistic and cultural practices; they are dealt with holistically, with little use for silos or binaries between social impact and cultural practice.

With obligations to family, community, and Country, First Nations theatre makers sustain a deep consideration of the politics and ethics of representing stories on the Australian stage. Since first contact and colonisation, representations of First Peoples in Australian discourse and media have been controlled, manipulated, and placed in the service of agendas to

[2] 'Cultural safety' is a term that originated in Aotearoa New Zealand nursing and healthcare (Papps and Ramsden 1996). It is now used in a range of Australian Aboriginal and Torres Strait Islander contexts (including arts and education) to denote creating environments that preserve, respect, value, and affirm the cultural identity, knowledge, and practices of First Nations peoples.

advance (White) settler domination and 'progress'. For the most part, these representations have vacillated between romanticised portrayals of primitivism and exotic 'otherness' and deficit-laden depictions of disadvantage that paint Aboriginal and Torres Strait Islander peoples as a 'problem' to be solved by White interventions and policies (Langton 1993). Writing a decade ago, Maryrose Casey (2013, 160–161) drew on Wesley Enoch's reflections to highlight how "there is a need to be aware of the image of Aboriginality that will be taken away by audience members who may well never either deal directly with Aboriginal people or see another Aboriginal performance." She went on to observe that artists such as Enoch must negotiate a "bind" between works that will invariably come to represent a "generalised notion of Indigenous people" to White audiences, but which are, in fact, expressions of "individual sensibility" (Casey 2013, 161). As Casey (2012, 2) writes elsewhere, on the mainstage, White audiences and producers have long played a role in determining "what is culturally real and unreal" in First Nations performance, based on notions of "authentic" representations of culture as being traditional, fixed, or archaic, rather than contemporary, fluid, and evolving (see also Thorner et al. 2018; Casey 2013). This attitude has shifted to some degree but persists today—with our observation that non-transformational trauma narratives have recently gained currency among mainstream (White) audiences as an expected benchmark for 'authentic' black theatre.

Nevertheless, contemporary theatre makers continually strive to challenge reductive representations of Aboriginal and Torres Strait Islander identity and culture and to bring their experiences and perspectives to audiences in all their complexity and nuance. A crucial facet of presenting such stories is finding empowering aesthetic frames through which to acknowledge and challenge the traumas, injustices, and oppressions that continue to impact Aboriginal and Torres Strait Islanders' lives in colonised Australia. Contemporary theatre makers have approached this in a variety of ways over the years, tackling difficult themes such as the Stolen Generations, intergenerational poverty, incarceration, and family violence through the prism of strength and survival (Casey and Craigie 2011). In discussing the integration of traditional dance and movement practices into contemporary performances, for example, Syron (2021, 102) suggests that a radical space of performative dialogue emerges—one that conveys the complexity of contemporary Indigenous lives:

> Through dance and movement the theatre makers were involved in connecting with wounds, losses, traumas, and memories carried by Indigenous bodies, whilst at the same time actively moving towards the restoration and celebration of the Indigenous body as a knowing subject.

This "restoration and celebration" of bodies enacts sovereignty over the stage and over the contemporary cultural landscape, challenging the preconceptions and prejudices of mainstream audiences. Also critical to this assertion of power and sovereignty in First Nations theatre is the use of humour in undercutting the traumas and indignities of life under colonisation. In her survey of Aboriginal and Torres Strait Islander monodramas, Casey (2013, 163) observed that humour and self-mockery were a common feature, "Enab[ling] people to survive and continue with some sense of self and dignity." We discuss later how humour is crucial to the health education works, which builds on millennia of yarning and storytelling practices that feature it as vital to entertainment, communication, and pedagogy.

Contemporary First Nations dramaturgies therefore have a strong legacy of deploying a complex array of traditional and contemporary approaches to tackle difficult themes. As Kabir Matharu (2009) observes from a medical humanities perspective, many Australian First Nations plays can be seen as instructive for healthcare professionals, exposing existing structural health inequities and depicting the erosion of social determinants of health and wellbeing. Jacob Boehme's *Blood on the Dancefloor* (2016) represents a significant recent work that addresses shame, stigma, and sexual health from a First Nations perspective. Produced by Ilbijerri, Boehme's ground-breaking performance integrated contemporary dance, digital media, and personal narrative to depict the experience of being Aboriginal, gay, and HIV positive. Made for public audiences, the work did not have an educational focus but instead was an intense celebration of hope, life, and love that surfaced a largely hidden issue facing many First Nations peoples today. Boehme described his approach as "such a different take on the HIV conversation to date—being very irreverent and very dark, black humour" (Campbell and Graffam 2018, 352). Through the work, Boehme explores themes of community, kinship, vulnerability, and acceptance through a story that might otherwise be mired in sorrow: "Here's another story that's about living and thriving, … rather than the usual AIDS plague where everyone dies. We live with it now. Our communities have been part of the fight dealing with HIV/AIDS since the

80s" (Boehme, interviewed by Bergman 2019). The work therefore has strong emotional, political, social, and cultural underpinnings, framed through a sense of resistance, survival, and celebration. Although intentionally educational, Kamarra's approach to the health works for Ilbijerri aligns strongly with this sensibility. As such, Boehme's work forms a kind of conceptual bridge we might cross between contemporary First Nations performance and theatre for health education. While First Nations contemporary theatre in Australia has always been concerned with promoting the strength, survival, and wellbeing of Aboriginal and Torres Strait Islander communities, we now turn towards a brief survey of theatre and performing arts used explicitly in health promotion and education in First Nations and global majority communities.

Theatre and Health Education: First Nations and Global Majority Approaches

The health education works discussed in this volume have been developed and toured in the context of intergenerational social and health inequities in Australia brought about by colonisation and sustained systemic racism across the intergovernmental domains of education, justice, social welfare, and health. This has resulted in Aboriginal and Torres Strait Islander peoples being disproportionately affected by poverty, disadvantage, illness, and low life expectancy, with efforts towards "closing the gap" between Aboriginal and Torres Strait Islander and non-Indigenous health outcomes failing to achieve results in many areas (see Commonwealth of Australia 2022). Aboriginal and Torres Strait Islander peoples have been identified as experiencing disproportionally higher rates of blood-borne viruses (BBV) and sexually transmissible infections (STIs) when compared with the non-Indigenous population (D'Costa et al. 2019). Despite Ilbijerri's longstanding efforts in this space through the productions *Chopped Liver* (2006–2009, 2017), *Body Armour* (2010–2013), *North West of Nowhere* (2014–2016), and *Viral—Are You the Cure?* (2018/2019), the Australian Federal Government (2018) recently identified a lack of culturally respectful health education and prevention services and the presence of shame and stigma as among many contributing factors to the disproportionate risks and burden of blood-borne viruses (BBV) and sexually transmissible infections (STI). This disparity, along with an alarming resurgence of syphilis in Aboriginal and Torres Strait Islander communities (Hui et al. 2022), led to the Victorian Department of Health's funding for Ilbijerri to develop *The Score*, which addresses sexual health and healthy relationships for young people. Strobel and Ward (2012) observe that Aboriginal and Torres Strait Islander peoples have experienced centuries of violence in relation to sexual health, including medical incarceration in "lock hospitals"[3] and medical experimentation. This is critical to understanding the fear, shame, and stigma that are associated with sexual health and BBV in this context. The issue of family violence (as addressed through the production *Scar Trees*) similarly disproportionately affects First Nations communities in Australia, with a lack of resources and high levels of shame and stigma also contributing to the challenge of providing support services (Fiolet et al. 2021). This speaks to Kamarra's intentional approach to challenging fear, shame, and stigma through health education theatre works.

First Nations-led approaches to health and wellbeing have continued to place their communities, cultures, and knowledges at the centre of efforts to address health and wellbeing inequities, with an identified need to adopt holistic, culturally led, strengths based approaches and to examine how *cultural* as well as social determinants of health might be considered in health promotion and prevention strategies (Dudgeon et al. 2020; Gee et al. 2014; Sunderland et al. 2023; Verbunt et al. 2021). An emerging body of evidence supports community-led, arts-based programs for health promotion and education in response to health inequities among Aboriginal and Torres Strait Islander communities in Australia (Hickey et al. 2021; McEwan et al. 2013; Sunderland et al. 2023). These approaches have been found to reduce stigma and increase capacity for open discussion around sensitive topics such as sexual health, create enjoyment and community connection in rural/remote regions, and can act as a catalyst for further work in prevention and harm minimisation (see Cairnduff et al. 2015; Rogers 2013). The imperative to adopt First Nations- and culturally led approaches to health education and promotion has contributed to Victoria's Department of Health engaging Ilbijerri to deliver this work since 2006 (see Victorian Government 2022).

While evidence is growing for the use of various art forms such as music, hip-hop, dance, and visual art in Aboriginal and Torres Strait Islander health promotion and education (see, for example, Anthony et al. 2018;

[3] "Lock hospitals" were secure facilities (prisons) where Aboriginal and Torres Strait Islanders Peoples were incarcerated during the nineteenth and twentieth centuries for having suspected "venereal disease" (see Pervan et al. 2020).

Cairnduff et al. 2015; McEwan et al. 2013), there is very little documentation or evaluation in applied theatre or theatre for health education in Australian First Nations contexts. An examination of productions entered into the AusStage database[4] yielded examples such as *The Kangaroo Tale* (1995) and its sequel *Slow Down Cuz* (1997), both Handspan Theatre Company shows incorporating puppetry, presented by the Koori Health Unit, and tackling sexual health and sex education; *Lost and Found in the Smoke* (2012), a school touring show by Ngarrama Productions about the dangers of smoking; and *Gift of Life* (2012), a show about kidney disease and organ donation, written by Ben Graetz, supported by the then Australian Government Organ and Tissue Authority, and toured by Artback Northern Territory throughout remote communities (see https://youtu.be/NvAKeMr2l6Y). Details about these examples are somewhat thin but demonstrate that this approach certainly is not new. More recently, JUTE Theatre Company in Far North Queensland, through its Dare to Dream program, includes touring works for children written by Isaac Drandic that address personal safety (*I Gut This Feeling* 2023) and road safety (*Back on Track* 2021–2023). Multi-art performances and festivals are often presented to coincide with annual events such as Mental Health Week and NAIDOC[5] week, where local Aboriginal Community Controlled Health Organisations (ACCHOs) are present to hand out information and provide health checks.

A review of scholarly literature for this study uncovered only a few theatre- or drama-based health education works in Aboriginal and Torres Strait Islander communities beyond the Ilbijerri works described in this volume. Fagan et al. (2015) discuss the Kasa Por Yarn (KPY) radio drama project (in English: "Just for a Chat"), which ran in the Torres Strait from 2010 to 2012. This aimed to raise awareness of HIV and STIs, building on and responding to community learning as a result of previous health initiatives in the area, including the Torres Hip Hop Project (McEwan et al. 2013). With the support of a Torres Strait Islander scriptwriter, the community developed KPY as a relationship drama about family and life in remote areas. The play was written and performed in the language of

[4] AusStage is a national database of live performance in Australia with entries going back to 1789: https://www.ausstage.edu.au/ausstage/pages/browse/

[5] NAIDOC originally stood for National Aborigines and Islanders Day Observance Committee, with NAIDOC week now a significant annual celebration of Aboriginal and Torres Strait Islander culture and achievements in Australia.

Yumpla Tok Kriol by local Torres Strait Islander performers. The authors discuss improvements in sexual health knowledge as a result of the project and offer reflections from community members on its value. Additionally, in the Torres Strait Islands and Far North Queensland, Mooney and Sariago (2015) discuss the 2Sprits program, a multi-arts HIV/AIDS whole-of-community education program that incorporated work with young people through the superhero characters "Condoman" and "Lubelicious" and the production of radio scripts that the authors note were a powerful tool to reach remote communities.

Globally, there is increasing evidence to support the effectiveness of theatre in health education, particularly in global majority and First Nations contexts, where it is commonly focused on HIV/AIDS and sexual health and includes projects in India, the USA, Africa, Indigenous and First Nations Canada, and Asia Pacific (Brodzinski 2010; Cahill 2017; Goulet et al. 2011; Haseman et al. 2014; Jaganath et al. 2014; Low 2020; Van Hout et al. 2020; Wells 2013). These projects adopt a range of approaches to theatre and performance, target various groups as participants and audiences, and represent a diversity of models in terms of funding and structure. Research into this work has highlighted the benefits of theatre and drama in promoting positive attitudes and behaviours, empowering people to explore complex emotional and social terrain through the art form, creating space for open dialogue and discussion, and reducing stigma in relation to sexual health (Goulet et al. 2011; Heard et al. 2019; Kauli 2018). Crucially, some projects were seen to provide an opportunity for communities to discuss inequities in healthcare systems and other legacies of colonial power (Flicker et al. 2014; Linds et al. 2013).

Despite growing evidence for the success of such programs, some tensions and challenges remain—both for program delivery and for measuring impact. The research has begun to highlight some lessons as to the pitfalls of theatre for health education, alongside what might represent best practice in terms of creating, delivering, and evaluating this work. As Katharine Low (2017) points out, this tension originates in how communities define concepts such as "health" and "wellbeing" and whether these are driven by Western models of an absence of disease or a notion of wellbeing that promotes neoliberal notions of productivity and market values. Cahill (2017) cautions against a focus on behaviour change at the individual level through individual storylines rather than addressing the structural inequities and social and cultural determinants of health. This places the burden on the individual and eliminates the opportunity for engaging participants with agency around the issues they face as a community. While encouraging behaviour change may certainly achieve positive outcomes in the short term, it is unlikely to have lasting effects. This can create tensions around evaluating the efficacy of programs, which can be difficult to achieve in a longitudinal sense and is still often undertaken using more traditional positivist approaches that privilege quantitative, longitudinal data as being the gold standard and therefore able to speak more effectively to the mainstream fields of medicine and social sciences—and by extension to government policymaking. However, as discussed by many in the field—particularly those working in First Nations health—this is not necessarily the most effective approach for evaluating arts-led, community-led practices (Brodzinski 2010; Keating 2009; Low 2017).

According to our review of the literature, the most effective programs are developed from the ground up with communities so that their own definitions of health and wellbeing, determined by cultural and social traditions, become the drivers for program goals and outputs (Low 2017). Katharine Low (2017) proposes that theatre and performance practice can offer ways of situating and articulating experiences of health that are relational to the individual, according to that person's own understandings of what health means, as shifting, transitional, and affective. Cultural understandings, material conditions, and emotions can contribute to a holistic model of what health "is" at any one time, to any one community and individual. Key strengths in these programs when done well include engaging audiences in active learning as opposed to top-down messaging; audiences see themselves reflected in the performers, storylines, and cultural content; projects typically adopt a whole-of-community approach that draws together target groups, stakeholders, community-controlled health organisations, and community leaders/Elders; the presence of peer mentoring and peer teaching within programs (Brodzinski 2010; Baxter and Low 2017; Cahill 2017). As will be discussed later, these notions of best practice have been implicitly present to varying degrees throughout Ilbijerri's health education works, driven largely by Kamarra's educational background, artistic instincts, and cultural positionality (as opposed to formal theoretical knowledge of theatre for health education). Certain elements, such as greater community engagement, were high on Kamarra's agenda for future iterations of the work. Of particular interest to us are those theatre- or drama-based programs for health education that are developed and delivered by established local theatre/performance companies. The Life Drama project in Papua New Guinea, for example, enabled the prodigious expertise and legacy of an existing company (Raun Raun) to be deployed for HIV/AIDS education in communities, thereby foregrounding localised cultural and aesthetic approaches to the issue and building a sustainable model for subsequent work into the future (Haseman et al. 2014).

Conclusion

In this chapter, we have offered an integrated examination of contemporary First Nations dramaturgies in Australia and theatre and drama as explicitly used for health education in First Nations and global majority contexts. The aim has been to locate our study of Ilbijerri's health education productions within a theoretical framework that encompasses theatre, performance, cultural practice, and holistic, arts-led approaches to health wellbeing in Aboriginal and Torres Strait Islander communities. This framework also represents an intersection between our disciplines as authors and collaborators, providing a grounding for the chapters that follow. We now move to the findings of our study, which illuminate three prominent themes across the works. The first of these, as discussed in the next chapter, focuses on culturally led, culturally safe practices both in creative development and performance of theatre for health education in a First Nations Australian context.

References

A Nightime Travesty. 2023. Devised and performed by Kamarra Bell-Wykes and Carly Shepperd (A Daylight Connection). Meat Market, Melbourne, Victoria, May 10–13, 2023.

Anthony, Brendan, Donna Weston, and Samuel Vallen. 2018. Thumbs Up: The Effective Use of Music in Health and Well-being Education for Australian Aboriginal Youth in Remote Communities. *International Journal of Community Music* 11 (1): 71–89. https://doi.org/10.1386/ijcm.11.1.71_1.

Australian Government. 2018. *Fifth National Aboriginal and Torres Strait Islander Blood Borne Viruses and Sexually Transmissible Infections Strategy 2018–2022*. Department of Health and Aged Care. https://www1.health.gov.au/internet/main/publishing.nsf/Content/ohp-bbvs-1/$File/ATSI-Fifth-Nat-Strategy-2018-22.pdf

Back on Track. 2021. By Isaac Drandic. Directed by Isaac Drandic. Produced by JUTE Theatre Company. Toured throughout Far North Queensland, April–June 2021.

Baxter, Veronica, and Katharine E. Low, eds. 2017. *Applied Theatre: Performing Health and Wellbeing*. London: Bloomsbury Methuen Drama. https://doi.org/10.5040/9781472584601.

Bergman, Gabi. 2019. Jacob Boehme on his Autobiographical *Blood on the Dancefloor*. *Aussietheatre.com*, July 30. https://www.aussietheatre.com.au/news/jacob-boehme-on-his-autobiographical-blood-on-the-dance-floor

Blood on the Dancefloor. 2016. By Jacob Boehme. Directed by Isaac Drandic. Produced by Ilbijerri Theatre Company. Arts Centre Melbourne, Melbourne, Victoria, August 20–21, 2016.

Boehme, Jacob. 2018. Keynote Address at the Australian Performing Arts Market 2018. Reproduced by Blackdance, August 7, 2019. https://www.blakdance.org.au/media-releases/jacob-boehme-keynote-address-at-australian-performing-arts-market-2018

Bracknell, Clint, Kylie Bracknell, Susan Fenty Studham, and Luzita Fereday. 2021. Supporting the performance of Noongar language in *Hecate*. *Theatre, Dance and Performance Training* 12 (3): 377–395. https://doi.org/10.1080/19443927.2021.1943506.

Brodzinski, Emma. 2010. *Theatre in Health and Care*. Springer International Publishing.

Cahill, Helen. 2017. Performing the Solution: Cautions and Possibilities When Using Theatre Conventions within HIV Prevention Programs. In *Applied Theatre: Performing Health and Wellbeing*, ed. Veronica Baxter and Katharine Low, 145–166. London: Bloomsbury Methuen Drama. https://doi.org/10.5040/9781472584601.ch-006.

Cairnduff, Sallie, Darren Braun, and Kaylie Harrison. 2015. HIV Free Generation: AH&MRC Street Art Project. *HIV Australia* 13 (3): 56–59. https://www.afao.org.au/wp-content/uploads/2017/03/HIVA-13-3-Fire_in_the_Belly.pdf.

Campbell, Alyson, and Jonathan Graffam. 2018. Blood, Shame, Resilience and Hope: Indigenous Theatre Maker Jacob Boehme's *Blood on the Dance Floor*. In *Viral Dramaturgies: HIV and AIDS in Performance in the Twenty-First Century*, ed. Alyson Campbell and Dirk Gindt, 343–365. Springer International Publishing.

Casey, Maryrose. 2000. From the Wings to Centre Stage: A Production Chronology of Theatre and Drama Texts by Indigenous Australian Writers. *Australasian Drama Studies* 37: 85–98. https://search.informit.org/doi/abs/10.3316/ielapa.200107835.

———. 2012. Colonisation, Notions of Authenticity and Aboriginal Australian Performance. *Critical Race and Whiteness Studies* 8 (1): 1–18.

———. 2013. Bold, Black, and Brilliant: Aboriginal Australian Drama. In *A Companion to Australian Aboriginal Literature*, ed. Belinda Wheeler, 155–172. Boydell & Brewer. http://www.jstor.org/stable/10.7722/j.ctt31njb6.15=Copy.

Casey, Maryrose, and Cathy Craigie. 2011. A Brief History of Indigenous Australian Contemporary Theatre. *Australian Script Centre.* https://australianplays.org/assets/files/resource/doc/2012/06/BlakStage_Essay_ABriefHistory_DUPL_1.pdf

Chase. 2022. By Carly Shepperd and Kamarra Bell-Wykes (A Daylight Connection). Directed by Kamarra Bell-Wykes. Malthouse, Melbourne, Victoria, March 16–20, 2022.

Commonwealth of Australia. 2022. *Commonwealth Closing the Gap Annual Report 2022.* National Indigenous Australians Agency. Canberra. https://www.niaa.gov.au/resource-centre/indigenous-affairs/commonwealth-closing-gap-annual-report-2022

D'Costa, Belinda, Roanna Lobo, Jessica Thomas, and James Steven Ward. 2019. Evaluation of the Young Deadly Free Peer Education Training Program: Early Results, Methodological Challenges, and Learnings for Future Evaluations. *Frontiers in Public Health* 7: 74. https://doi.org/10.3389/fpubh.2019.00074.

Dudgeon, Pat, Abigail Bray, Dawn Darlaston-Jones, and Roz Walker 2020. Aboriginal Participatory Action Research: An Indigenous Research Methodology Strengthening Decolonisation and Social and Emotional Wellbeing. Discussion Paper. Melbourne: The Lowitja Institute. https://www.lowitja.org.au/page/services/resources/Cultural-and-social-determinants/mental-health/aboriginal-participatory-action-research-an-indigenous-research-methodology-strengthening-decolonisation-and-social-and-emotional-wellbeing

Enoch, Wesley. 2002. "Why Do We Applaud?" In *The 7 Stages of Grieving* (3rd edition), by Wesley Enoch and Deborah Mailman, 13–16. Playlab Press.

Fagan, Patricia S., Heather K. Robertson, Alisa E. Pedrana, Alexandra Raulli, and Alan A. Crouch. 2015. Successes in Sexual Health Communications Development, Programmatic Implementation and Evaluation in the Torres Strait Region 2006 to 2012. *Australian and New Zealand Journal of Public Health* 39 (3): 270–276. https://onlinelibrary.wiley.com/doi/epdf/10.1111/1753-6405.12356.

Fiolet, Renee, Laura Tarzia, Mohajer Hameed, and Kelsey Hegarty. 2021. Indigenous Peoples' Help-Seeking Behaviors for Family Violence: A Scoping Review. *Trauma, Violence, & Abuse* 22 (2): 370–380. https://doi.org/10.1177/1524838019852638.

Flicker, Sarah, Jessica Yee Danforth, Ciann Wilson, Vanessa Oliver, June Larkin, Jean-Paul Restoule, Claudia Mitchell, Erin Konsmo, Randy Jackson, and Tracey Prentice. 2014. 'Because we have Really Unique Art': Decolonizing Research with Indigenous Youth Using the Arts. *International Journal of Indigenous Health* 1 (01): 16–34. https://doi.org/10.18357/ijih.101201513271.

Gee, Graham, Pat Dudgeon, Clinton Schultz, Amanda Hart, and Kerrie Kelly. 2014. Aboriginal and Torres Strait Islander social and emotional wellbeing. In

Working Together: Aboriginal and Torres Strait Islander Mental Health and Wellbeing Principles and Practice, ed. Pat Dudgeon, Helen Milroy, and Roz Walker, 55–68. Canberra: Commonwealth of Australia.

Gilbert, Kevin. 1988. *The Cherry Pickers: The First Written Aboriginal Play*. Canberra: Burrambinga Books.

Goulet, Linda, Warren Linds, Jo-Ann Episkenew, and Karen Schmidt. 2011. Creating a Space for Decolonization: Health Through Theatre with Indigenous Youth. *Native Studies Review* 20 (1): 89–116. http://publications.usask.ca/nativestudiesreview/.

Harvey, Margaret. 2018. *Woer Wayepa-the Water is Rising*: A Torres Strait Islander Approach to Knowledge Mobilisation, and Saibaian Approach to Cultural Knowledge Transference to Performative Storytelling. *Australasian Drama Studies* 73: 160–185. https://search.informit.org/doi/10.3316/ielapa.146628555647362.

Haseman, Brad, Andrea Baldwin, and Hayley Linthwaite. 2014. Folk Opera: Stories Crossing Borders in Papua New Guinea. *RiDE: The Journal of Applied Theatre and Performance* 19 (1): 98–109. https://doi.org/10.1080/13569783.2013.872430.

Heard, Emma, Lisa Fitzgerald, Sina Vaai, Maxine Whittaker, Tonumaipe'a J. Aiolupotea, Fiona Collins, and Allyson Mutch. 2019. Intimate Partner Violence Prevention: Using Interactive Drama for Intimate Relationship Education with Young People in Samoa. *Sex Education* 19 (6): 691–705. https://doi.org/10.1080/14681811.2019.1597697.

Hickey, Sophie, Yvette Roe, Caroline Harvey, Sue Kruske, Anton Clifford-Motopi, Ike Fisher, Brenna Bernardino, and Sue Kildea. 2021. Community-Based Sexual and Reproductive Health Promotion and Services for First Nations People in Urban Australia. *International Journal of Women's Health 2021* (13): 467–478. https://doi.org/10.2147/IJWH.S297479.

Hui, Ben B., James S. Ward, Rebecca Guy, Matthew G. Law, Richard T. Gray, and David G. Regan. 2022. Impact of Testing Strategies to Combat a Major Syphilis Outbreak Among Australian Aboriginal and Torres Strait Islander Peoples: A Mathematical Modeling Study. *Open Forum Infectious Diseases* 9 (5, ofac119): 1–8. https://doi.org/10.1093/ofid/ofac119.

Hyland, Nicola, Liza-Mare Syron, and Maryrose Casey. 2018. 'Turangawaewae': A Place to Stand in Contemporary Indigenous Performance in Australasia and Beyond. *Australasian Drama Studies* 73: 1–16. https://search.informit.org/doi/10.3316/informit.146442225934780.

I Gut This Feeling. 2023. By Isaac Drandic. Directed by Ian Wilkes. Produced by JUTE Theatre Company. Toured throughout Far North Queensland, July-September 2023.

Ilbijerri Theatre Company. n.d. Social Impact Program. Accessed June 21, 2023. https://www.ilbijerri.com.au/programs/social-impact-program/

Jaganath, D., C. Mulenga, R.M. Hoffman, J. Hamilton, and G. Boneh. 2014. This is My Story: Participatory Performance for HIV and AIDS Education at the University of Malawi. *Health Education Research* 29 (4): 554–565. https://doi.org/10.1093/her/cyt074.

Kauli, Jacqueline. 2018. Awareness Community Theatre: A Local Response to HIV and AIDS in Papua New Guinea. In *Viral Dramaturgies: HIV and AIDS in Performance in the Twenty-First Century*, ed. Alyson Campbell and Dirk Gindt. Springer International Publishing.

Keating, Clare. 2009. *'Chopped Liver' Evaluation Report. Effective Change Pty Ltd*. Melbourne: Ilbijerri Theatre Company. Supplied.

Kelly, Kathryn, and Emily Coleman. 2019. Community Engagement in Independent Performance-Making in Australia: A Case Study of *Rovers*. *Social Alternatives* 38 (1): 53–64. https://search.informit.org/doi/abs/10.3316/ielapa.340113329192511.

Langton, Marcia. 1993. Well, I Saw it on the Television and I Heard it on the Radio. Sydney: Australian Film Commission. https://www-austlit-edu-au.eu1.proxy.openathens.net/austlit/page/C727650

Linds, Warren, Heather Ritenburg, Linda Goulet, Jo-Ann Episkenew, Karen Schmidt, Nuno Ribeiro, and Allison Whiteman. 2013. Layering Theatre's Potential for Change: Drama, Education, and Community in Aboriginal Health Research. *Canadian Theatre Review* 154: 37–43. https://doi.org/10.3138/CTR.154.007.

Lo, Jacqueline, and Helen Gilbert. 2002. Toward a Topography of Cross-Cultural Theatre Praxis. *TDR* 46 (3): 31–53. http://www.jstor.org/stable/1146995.

Low, Katharine E. 2017. Understanding Health, Wellbeing, the Millennium Development Goals and Health Inequities. In *Applied Theatre: Performing Health and Wellbeing*, ed. Veronica Baxter and Katharine E. Low, 11–40. London: Bloomsbury Methuen Drama. https://doi.org/10.5040/9781472584601.ch-001.

———. 2020. *Applied Theatre and Sexual Health Communication: Apertures of Possibility*. London: Palgrave Macmillan.

Malthouse Theatre. 2023. Chase. Accessed August 14, 2023. https://www.malthousetheatre.com.au/tickets/malthouse-theatre/chase-2023/

Matharu, Kabir. 2009. Using Indigenous Australian Drama to Break Cultural Barriers in Healthcare Relationships. *Medical Humanities* 45 (1): 47–53. https://doi.org/10.1136/jmh.2008.000364.

McEwan, Alexandra, Alan Crouch, Heather Robertson, and Patricia Fagan. 2013. The Torres Indigenous Hip Hop Project: Evaluating the Use of Performing Arts as a Medium for Sexual Health Promotion. *Health Promotion Journal of Australia* 24 (2): 132–136. https://doi.org/10.1071/HE12924.

Mooney, Brett, and Phillip Sariago. 2015. 2Spirits: Providing a Multi-Generational, Culturally Competent Approach to Health Promotion for Aboriginal and

Torres Strait Islander Communities. *HIV Australia* 13 (3): 34–35. https://www.afao.org.au/wp-content/uploads/2017/03/HIVA-13-3-Fire_in_the_Belly.pdf.

Nair, Sonia, Jessica Nicholas, Cher Tan, Barney Zwartz, Cameron Woodhead, and Mahmood Fazal. 2023. The Play that Asks: What Happens When Love Politics and Racism Collide? A Review of *A Nightime Travesty*, Performed by Kamarra Bell-Wykes and Carly Shepperd. *The Age*, May 11. https://www.theage.com.au/culture/theatre/christos-tsiolkas-loaded-has-finally-hit-the-stage-but-is-it-good-20230511-p5d7nd.html

Nakata, Martin. 2007. The Cultural Interface. *The Australian Journal of Indigenous Education* 36 (S1): 7–14. https://doi.org/10.1017/S1326011100004646.

Neumeier, Beate. 2014. Performative Lives—Transformative Practices: Wesley Enoch and Deborah Mailman, *The 7 Stages of Grieving*, and Richard Frankland, *Conversations with the Dead*. In *Decolonizing the Landscape*, ed. Beate Neumeier and Kay Schaffer, 275–292. Rodopi. https://doi.org/10.1163/9789401210423_016.

Papps, Elaine, and Irihapeti Ramsden. 1996. Cultural Safety in Nursing: The New Zealand Experience. *International Journal for Quality in Health Care* 8 (5): 491–497. https://doi.org/10.1093/intqhc/8.5.491.

Perkins, June. 2000. 7 Valleys of Nurturing: Exploring the Performing Arts Philosophy of Wesley Enoch: A Profile. *Australasian Drama Studies* 37: 18–26. https://search.informit.org/doi/abs/10.3316/ielapa.200107828.

Pervan, Jade, Kathleen Musulin, and Bob Dorey. 2020. The Path of Pain: A Case Study in Understanding Trauma, Acknowledging Truth and Enabling Healing Through the Bernier and Dorre Islands Lock Hospital Histories. *Historic Environment* 32 (2): 90–106. https://search.informit.org/doi/abs/10.3316/informit.831887652954388.

Prendergast, Monica, and Juliana Saxton, eds. 2016. *Applied Theatre: International Case Studies and Challenges for Practice (Second Edition)*. Intellect Books.

Rogers, Matthew. 2013. Connecting with Youth: How arts-based health campaigns are engaging young Aboriginal people in NSW. *HIV Australia* 11 (3): 46–48. https://www.afao.org.au/publications/hiv-australia/hiv-australia-2013/.

Strobel, Natalie A., and James Ward. 2012. Education Programs for Indigenous Australians about Sexually Transmitted Infections and Bloodborne Viruses. Resource sheet no. 14. Canberra: Australian Institute of Health and Welfare and Australian Institute of Family Studies. https://www.aihw.gov.au/getmedia/00250e14-7b83-4da8-994e-723a25d96ab7/ctgc-rs14.pdf.aspx?inline=true

Sunderland, Naomi, Phil Graham, Brydie-Leigh Bartleet, Darren Garvey, Clint Bracknell, Kristy Apps, Glenn Barry, Rae Cooper, Brigitta Scarfe, and Stacey Vervoort. 2023. First Nations Music as a Determinant of Health in Australia and Vanuatu: Political and Economic Determinants. *Health Promotion International* 38, no. 2: daac190. https://doi.org/10.1093/heapro/daac190.

Syron, Liza-Mare. 2021. *Rehearsal Practices of Indigenous Women Theatre Makers.* Springer International Publishing.

Thorner, Sabra, Fran Edmonds, Maree Clarke, and Paola Balla. 2018. Maree's Backyard: Intercultural Collaborations for Indigenous Sovereignty in Melbourne. *Oceania* 88 (3): 269–291. https://doi.org/10.1002/ocea.5206.

Thurow, Susan. 2018. *Namatjira*: Beyond the Script—Visual and Performative Aesthetics as Conduits for the Communication of Western Aranda Ontology. *Australasian Drama Studies* 73: 130–159. https://search.informit.org/doi/abs/10.3316/ielapa.146609922676104.

Van Hout, Marie Claire, Rosemary Mhlanga-Gunda, and Stephanie Kewley. 2020. Using Performance and Theatre Arts in HIV Interventions and HIV Programming in Sub-Saharan Africa: A Scoping Review of Extant Literature. *Journal of Sustainable Development Africa* 21 (4): 178–213. https://jsd-africa.com/Jsda/2019%20V21%20No4%20Winter/article21-04.html.

Verbunt, Ebony, Joanne Luke, Yin Paradies, Muriel Bamblett, Connie Salamone, Amanda Jones, and Margaret Kelaher. 2021. Cultural Determinants of Health for Aboriginal and Torres Strait Islander People–a Narrative Overview of Reviews. *International Journal for Equity in Health* 20: 1–9. https://link.springer.com/article/10.1186/s12939-021-01514-2.

Victorian Government. 2022. *Victorian Aboriginal Sexual and Reproductive Health Plan 2022.* Victoria State Government Department of Health. https://www.health.vic.gov.au/publications/victorian-aboriginal-sexual-and-reproductive-health-plan-2022-30

Viral—Are You the Cure? 2018. By Maryann Sam. Directed by Kamarra Bell-Wykes. Various sites throughout Victoria, 2018–2019.

Wells, Trish. 2013. Insights into Approaching Sexual Health Education Through Applied Theatre Methodology. *Applied Theatre Research.* 1 (2): 203–215. https://doi.org/10.1386/atr.1.2.203_1.

Welsh, Blayne. 2018. The Hepatitis C Trilogy: A Case for Indigenous Theatre as a Contemporary Manifestation of Traditional Healing Business. *Australasian Drama Studies* 73: 20–41. https://search.informit.org/doi/abs/10.3316/ielapa.146479491877297.

Whose Gonna Love 'Em? I am that I AM. 2022. By Kamarra Bell-Wykes. Directed by Kamarra Bell-Wykes. Footscray Community Arts Centre, Melbourne, Victoria, November 23–27.

Wilson, Shawn. 2008. *Research is Ceremony: Indigenous Research Methods.* Fernwood.

Woodland, Sarah, Kamarra Bell-Wykes, and Carissa Lee Godwin. 2023. Yarning Up Relations: Enacting a Relational Ethics in Cross-Cultural Research-Based Theater. *Qualitative Inquiry* 29 (2): 393–402. https://doi.org/10.1177/10778004221099561.

CHAPTER 4

Culturally Led, Culturally Safe Performance Making

Abstract This chapter presents the first of the findings from our study into the five health education works led by Kamarra Bell-Wykes and produced by Ilbijerri Theatre Company from 2006 to 2019. These findings draw on interviews conducted with eight practitioners who were involved over the years as performers, production staff, and advisors, a research yarn conducted between co-authors Sarah and Kamarra, and Kamarra's own critical reflections while putting together this volume. We also analysed documents and data from Ilbijerri's corporate archive and published works such as those by Clare Keating (*'Chopped Liver' Evaluation Report*. Effective Change Pty Ltd. Melbourne: Ilbijerri Theatre Company. Supplied, 2009) and Blayne Welsh (The Hepatitis C Trilogy: A Case for Indigenous Theatre as a Contemporary Manifestation of Traditional Healing Business. *Australasian Drama Studies* 73: 20–41. https://search.informit.org/doi/abs/10.3316/ielapa.146479491877297, 2018). Here we discuss the first of four prominent themes within the data: the importance of culturally led, culturally safe approaches to making theatre in health education in the First Nations Australian context. This includes the importance of First Nations cultural leadership at every stage from conception through to production, performance, and touring; the need for meaningful community consultation and engagement; and the promotion of cultural safety through protocols and practices that honour the lived experience, cultural obligations, and 'colonial load' for creative

S. Woodland, K. Bell-Wykes, *First Nations Australian Theatre for Health Equity*, https://doi.org/10.1007/978-3-031-65506-7_4

teams. We argue that centring culture in these foundational ways is essential for the works to achieve their educational goals while also progressing the dramaturgies of wellbeing, strength, and resistance that characterise contemporary First Nations theatre in Australia.

Keywords First Nations theatre • Theatre in education • Applied theatre • Arts and health • Theatre for health education

In Australia and internationally, there is growing recognition that Indigenous and First Nations peoples are best placed to take control of those issues that disproportionately impact their communities; and that First Nations led initiatives that are strengths based and culturally focused are more likely to succeed in their goals of educating and empowering communities in relation to health and wellbeing (Dudgeon et al. 2020; Verbunt et al. 2021). Further, wellbeing is considered holistically as encompassing cultural resilience, empowerment, agency, and self-determination (Gee et al. 2014). This includes the importance of cultural leadership at every stage from conception through to production, performance, and touring; the inclusion of community-led, community-engaged practices from the ground up; and the promotion of cultural safety through protocols and practices that honour the lived experience, cultural obligations, and 'colonial load' for creative teams. As Liza-Mare Syron (2021, 79) states, contemporary Indigenous theatre (albeit drawing from Western performance forms) is a cultural practice: "Performance is a culturally charged medium through which Indigenous peoples platform, express, and impart their cultural knowledge in a very public way." We argue that centring culture in these foundational ways is essential for the works to achieve their educational goals while also progressing the dramaturgies of wellbeing, strength, and resistance that characterise contemporary First Nations theatre in Australia as discussed in the previous chapter (Figs. 4.1 and 4.2).

First Nations Cultural Leadership

The strength of the health education theatre works discussed here lies first and foremost in being designed and delivered by Ilbijerri, one of Australia's longest running and most recognised First Nations contemporary performing arts companies. With Kamarra as the principal creative driver of

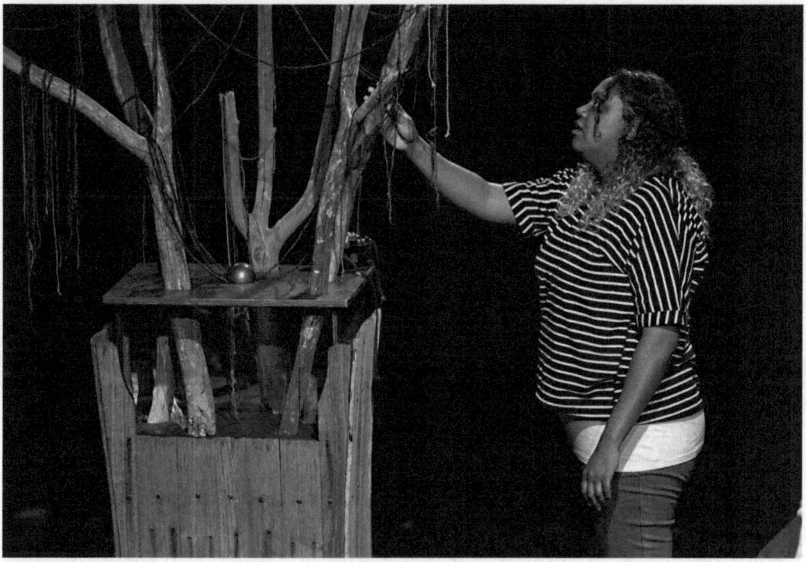

Fig. 4.1 Maurial Spearim, *Scar Trees*. Image by Tiffanie Garvie (2019)

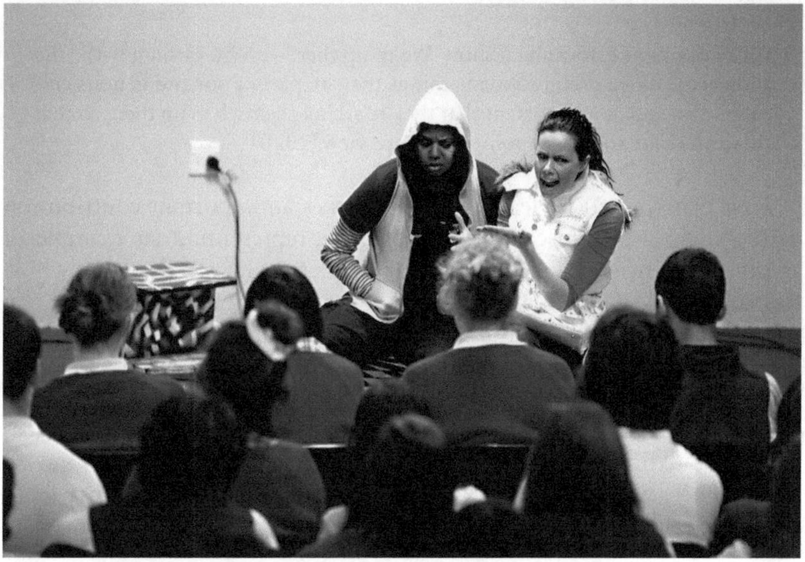

Fig. 4.2 Maurial Spearim (L) and Sandy Greenwood (R), *Body Armour* school performance. Image by James Henry (2011)

the works, production teams have been predominantly made up of established and emerging First Nations artists, with some support from non-Indigenous personnel. With the more recent production of *Viral—Are you the Cure?* all roles were filled by First Nations or persons of colour. The commissions for these works mostly came from the Victorian state Department of Health, which, while increasingly acknowledging the importance of Aboriginal and Torres Strait Islander approaches, still bases much of its delivery (and notably its evaluations) on Western models for health intervention, education, and promotion. Nevertheless, the content and approach to making the works were subsequently negotiated and honed by first and foremost privileging Aboriginal and Torres Strait Islander audiences and therefore centring cultural perspectives and practices. Some of the tensions and challenges inherent in this process are highlighted later, however, findings from the data point to the fact that this First Nations artistic leadership ensured that these works came from a place of cultural integrity and strength that were key to their success.

In his 2021 interview, Ngarigo health worker and artist Peter Waples-Crowe observed, "I think just it being Aboriginal led, and for Aboriginal communities makes it work." Performer Jesse Butler pointed out that this has an impact in terms of First Nations audiences seeing themselves reflected in the performances:

> We're not just performing a show. We're up there—we're yarning with [the audience]. We're doing so many things that are part of our Indigenous culture … because it's important that they're seeing themselves up there so that they can relate to what's going on. (Interview, 2020)

First Nations artistic leadership also makes an important contribution to the wider arts landscape in this country, representing an example of artistic excellence as explained by Peter Waples-Crowe: "I think the whole format, the way we're using health theatre as health promotion, an Aboriginal company, Aboriginal actors, Aboriginal writers, usually, and then Aboriginal health workers. So you know, we're showing the mainstream, this is how we do it, and innovation and ways to help promote. I'm just saying, it's good to bring Aboriginal excellence into White spaces as well, you know.

Audiences watching the early performances of *Chopped Liver* gave feedback that echoed these sentiments:

> It was really good to see some Indigenous performance, and as a Murri, here is a company willing to showcase our talents.
>
> Great to see a play set in a Nunga way of doing business. (Keating 2009, 16–17)

As suggested by these reflections, cultural leadership is vital in ensuring that there is ethical, appropriate, and inspiring representation of Aboriginal and Torres Strait Islander peoples and cultures on the stage, which in turn contributes to outcomes in health education and builds community strength and capacity as discussed in later chapters. The underpinning of First Nations leadership (and ownership) within these works operates as the essential bedrock for all that follows. It supports efforts towards decolonising the fields of both theatre and health and enacts sovereignty over how health and wellbeing knowledge is translated through culturally led contemporary performance.

Community Consultation and Engagement

To strengthen efforts towards decolonising and decentring practices, there is an identified need to engage in meaningful community consultation and collaboration so that works accurately and respectfully reflect the concerns of communities and will succeed in reaching those communities. This is not only considered best practice in terms of working in First Nations contexts but also reflects best practice in theatre for health promotion and education through theatre (Brodzinski 2010; Low 2020); and global health promotion scholarship more broadly, where the cultivation of community partnerships and capacity is seen as integral to achieving health education and promotion outcomes (Laverack and Mohammadi 2011). Alyson Campbell and Dirk Gindt (2018, 28) note in relation to theatre for HIV education, "This principle, that people directly affected by an issue should be central to discourses, actions and representations about them ('nothing about us without us'), is the key ethical basis and starting point for the creation of new performance work." In the five health education works discussed here, creative teams aimed to achieve this community accountability in three ways: through engaging with the reference group of health professionals and partners to inform the development of shows; through consultation and liaison with key community organisations, leaders, and Elders so that audiences would attend the performances and be given access to ongoing health advice and support afterwards; and through workshops where target communities and audiences had input into the development of shows. This last approach was introduced in *Viral* and developed further through *Scar Trees.*

As described in Chap. 2, a formal reference group was established for *Chopped Liver*, made up of professionals from the Department of Health (as principal funders), as well as other partners and stakeholders such as Victorian Aboriginal Community Controlled Health Organisation (VACCHO) and Hepatitis Victoria. This model continued through subsequent productions, drawing in members from other services and organisations depending on the topic being investigated. The purpose of the reference group was to give advice and guidance in relation to specific facts and information on health issues, technical language, the latest treatments, and an expert understanding of the barriers and enablers to healthy behaviours and seeking treatment. Kamarra acknowledged the value of the reference groups over the years, which had at times played a pivotal role in identifying significant elements that the creative teams may have missed.

> Sometimes they'll point out something that I haven't thought of that comes from their very specific detailed Community and health information that really helps to pivot a character in an even more empowering way. (Interview, 2021)

Some creative tensions arising from the reference groups' involvement are discussed later, however, they also provided important advocacy, support, and liaison in communities during tours. They linked the team in with local health workers, or joined tours themselves, to provide information to audiences after the shows. Kamarra therefore described the reference groups as "a multifunctioning health expert think tank … that would perform different roles across the life of the show." Kamarra did, however, come to realise that the reference group was only one part of the process of engaging with communities.

> Once we started performing - doing the yarning circles and getting community responses and particularly doing - performing in the prisons, I started to realise the real reference group for me was the yarning circles. It was the community's response. Those were the things that I was starting to use as my measures of success. …The reference group informs the work and … is the measuring stick along the way and then the audiences become the measure of success.

This realisation went on to inform Kamarra's developing approach post-*Chopped Liver*, which led towards deeper community engagement through workshops and participation as discussed below.

In addition to the reference group, the need for consultation and engagement with communities in advance of touring was seen as a vital cultural protocol to conducting healing business in a particular place and essential to achieving community buy-in that would increase the reach and impacts of works. This was achieved to varying degrees over the years, with interviewees acknowledging the importance of this but also how challenging it can be from a logistical perspective. Mary Quinsacara described community liaison as the "glue" that needs to be applied for there to be community buy-in and attendance (interview, 2020). Laila Thaker highlighted the importance of having "someone on the ground there within the community to be working on the project with you from the get-go" and building meaningful connections and relationships with them (interview, 2021). Although Laila acknowledged how this can be difficult to achieve sometimes, especially trying to do this in a non-Indigenous funding and touring framework:

> I think this is why working in the arts as a blackfulla is so difficult and whitefullas don't understand that either. It's like, well we're here trying to produce in a White structure, but actually it's tough man. We still need to be respectful of protocol and get the right permissions and stuff like that, but whitefullas don't understand that takes time.

Clare Keating's (2009, 19) report on *Chopped Liver* highlighted the need to take the time and find the correct partners and advocates within a community:

> Finding the 'right' person in the community is key to drawing a crowd. But there is no real formula for finding the 'right' person. Unfortunately, shows can be cancelled at the last minute or the team can turn up to put on a show for a very small audience, which can be frustrating if it is known that a larger audience could have been attracted with the right promotion or encouragement or better timing.

The need to consult with the 'right' people was evident in one of the *Viral* performances, where Kamarra and Mary Quinsacara recalled that the team drove an hour and a half to a community only to find just two health workers in the audience. Kamarra recalled asking them, "'Where is everybody? Where's the mob? Where's the community?' [and they said], 'Oh, they don't like coming to the school. It's not a culturally safe place for them,'" despite having initially chosen that performance space. Kamarra recalled that they had a few shows like that, which Mary observed was highly frustrating and disappointing for the touring ensemble. Nazaree Dickerson also related an anecdote that reflected this issue, where they had arrived in a community recently engaged in sorry business, which had led to a violent conflict within that community.

> It actually wasn't safe for us to be there. … I think it's important that there's connections made to find this information out. … With *Scar Trees*, I was talking to Aboriginal corporations and so I was speaking to their one community engagement officer. They don't necessarily know everything that's going on. (Interview, 2021)

She went on to suggest a multi-tiered approach to community liaison that would include community members at both the organisational and grassroots levels, "So that when you're sending a company in that they're aware if there's anything major going down, it's about safety on all parts, I think." Kamarra and Melodie Reynolds-Diarra echoed this sentiment in their conversation, where they agreed that successful community engagement was about more than just having a local health organisation representative on the ground, but also other key people in the community:

> Kamarra: Yes, you want somebody that's in the organisation that's hosting, but you need to have the Aunties in charge, or the fulla that's in charge inside [the prison] who's also a part of that engagement with that community.
>
> Melodie: Yeah, you find the most respected Elder or person in prison and you've got a mob behind them straightaway. (Interview, 2021)

As an example, Melodie recalled one prison performance of *Chopped Liver* where there had been no First Nations audience members in attendance until an incarcerated relative of fellow performer Isaac Drandic received word that he was in the performance, after which he rallied his peers to attend the show. The two went on to discuss how getting an audience to a show could be as simple as using the community or health service bus to go around and pick people up, thereby removing one of the barriers for attendance— "It's not rocket science," Kamarra said. Laila also acknowledged, "Unless someone's actually got a car or a van to go and pick up people, community engagement's hard." The simplicity of this solution was not lost on Kamarra, who has since advocated for this in more recent tours of *The Score*. Kamarra also identified a need for producers to have some interest or experience in community development practice, which would strengthen their capacity to cultivate the necessary relationships and maximise the impact of shows.

Kamarra's approach to community engagement evolved over the course of developing the works, so that by the time of *Viral,* in her role as an Education and Learning Manager at Ilbijerri, she recognised the need to engage more deeply with communities affected by the issues. *Viral* (written by Maryanne Sam) was greatly informed by the community workshops that Kamarra instigated to find out more about why Aboriginal and Torres Strait Islander peoples were not taking up the new treatment for hepatitis C. She later described how powerful this process had been, not only in terms of developing authentic content for the play but also providing a space for people to openly discuss their experiences for the first time.

> We found that through these yarning circles, we also had people though that were telling us things and confessing things and revealing things and connecting in a way about living with the virus and about their fears around the treatment and around the challenges with their broader lives that I - they said to us often that they had never shared these types of things or had these conversations. So we were just engaged in some of the most raw, soul-exposing conversations and really beautiful empowering conversations that we just pulled so much information from, that then went into the writing of the play. I just found that there were things that we discovered through those workshops that I never would have been able to myself make up as a writer and do justice to and that also though, that the workshops were so beneficial and effecting to the Community members that got to participate.

This level of community engagement created high levels of support for the show from community and prison audiences once it came to tour. Jesse Butler described how one workshop participant in prison had informed his character and storyline, leading to a strong sense of connection to the performance for that man and his peers and a conviction for Jesse that the process had been much deeper than just a theatre performance.

> You know, he came up to me afterwards and gave me a hug and thanked him for doing his story and stuff, and I was like, nothing can top this. It was just this moment of, 'What even am I doing right now?' … this isn't about theatre right now, this is just about connecting. … To actually see that connection and be a part of it, and to walk into a room where there are a bunch of prisoners or just people from the community centre that are worrying, going, 'What the hell is going on? I just came in for a cup of tea.' Then having this thing, just this connection that then you create, and then afterwards they're sitting around and actually able to open up in front of you. … All of a sudden it became about this connection that we had with people and the message I think was pretty clear … it was pretty impactful.

Kamarra related how this same participant had rejected the idea of seeking treatment during the development workshops, but attending the performance 18 months later, he told her that he had participated in the treatment and recently cleared the virus.

> I guess that, to me, was a testament that this was the track that we needed to keep going down and exploring and expanding. Even that was such a small thing, and it was like a year and a half these lads had waited for us to come back. After only two workshops and to see how much gratitude and appreciation and just the disbelief that we'd even come back and that we'd come back with something that was better than they thought.

The community workshops in *Scar Trees* (adapted from a script by Declan Furber Gillick) were conducted with young people in care to explore the issue of family violence from their perspective. These were less successful in terms of providing a sense of continuity from workshops to performance, however, Nazaree Dickerson recalled how those young people who did see the show "had a real sense of pride" in their contributions. These experiences of engaging with communities through workshops were formative for Kamarra's developing practice, ultimately leading to her idea for working long-term with communities to achieve more lasting engagement and transformative change through *The Score*.

Lived Experience and 'Colonial Load'

First Nations arts practitioners are charged with a huge weight of responsibility in terms of asserting ownership and leadership over projects in the face of mainstream structural resistance and engaging meaningfully with communities and stakeholders to deliver the work. In health and wellbeing-focused projects, they also often must do this while navigating complex social issues that directly affect their own communities (sometimes their own family members). This cultural load—or colonial load—can be difficult to carry without strong self-care practices and effective avenues for support and debriefing. As Bracknell et al. (2021) discuss in relation to creating the work *Hecate*, "Every stage of the production risked triggering trauma associated with colonisation and language loss" (385). This is true also of works that address the kinds of health and social inequities exemplified in Ilbijerri's Social Impact Program. In discussing her involvement as a community facilitator with *Scar Trees*, Nazaree Dickerson highlighted:

> [These are] hugely complex issues in our communities. There's no easy way to navigate them from one community to the next, from one family to the next. So, yeah, that's where a lot of that weight sits, I think, is the fact that they are so complex.

While performer Melodie Reynolds-Diarra spoke about this in terms of the healing work that the plays aim to achieve:

> If the play's there to heal, it's going to obviously bring up stuff in order to be healed. … That's, I suppose, why we do it in the first place is that we want to make a change from this, we want to bring stuff up into the - so that we can talk about it and if this horrific stuff was triggered by what we've said, there's chance for help now.

For Melodie, this meant having to "emotionally guard" herself, and shared a strong analogy for how she approached this:

> If someone's drowning in the water, you don't jump into that dangerous water with them because you're in it. … But if you look for a tool to be able to reach out to help them, or if you safely reach out to help them and stuff like that, that's the way there to pull them through. So, I made sure and not jump in the water with a lot of the stories. Sometimes they get you by surprise and you may have dreams or thoughts or feelings about that person a few days, or weeks, or months later, or something like that, or something could trigger it. But, same time, you just got to remember the initial 'why' you went into it, I suppose.

As explored later, much of the plays' success stemmed from the safe, stigma-free space that they opened for discussion about difficult issues, but this also came with some risks for the performers where, as Melodie pointed out, "Everyone feels like they can tell you stuff." She therefore emphasised the need for putting spiritual safeguards in place:

> Having a template or something energetic to put there like to guard your spirit … [from] what you may encounter, and the fact that there's I think a lot of people are going to be vulnerable to you but don't be vulnerable back.

In addition to the weight of the topics being covered in the plays, and the stories and experiences shared by audiences, the research showed a need to account for the different lived experiences of creative team members. Some interviewees had direct experience of the issues under exploration, or direct family or Mob connections with those affected (including incarcerated audience members), whereas others' experiences of the issues were more arm's length. Either way, most felt a strong impact, particularly from touring into prisons. Nazaree discussed parallels between the story in *Scar Trees* and her own lived experience:

> Look, I think for me, it comes from a place of lived experience. My own experience as a young person with domestic violence in my house, seeing things, going to visit people in prison that I wasn't necessarily fond of. A lot of personal memories attached to that, but also having grown up in community that is—it's very common to have a lot of family members in prison … I can't even count the amount of brother boys, cousins … and sister girls that I've got in jail right now. That's just kind of their life and so there is this—a little bit—a feeling of guilt because I actually was steered away from that. I luckily escaped that by the skin of my teeth, and it could have easily been me on that side. So, there's this element of going in there and not wanting to, yeah - not wanting to offend, but just being there out of love, because you understand. But, yeah, it's a strange feeling. It is, actually, a really strange feeling, but very rewarding and such an honour to do, because the - the response you get is always amazing.

Nazaree's account points towards the complexities of, on the one hand, having lived experience that raised difficult feelings and, on the other hand, how this deepened her sense of "honour" in addressing the issues and giving back to the community. Melodie Reynolds-Diarra echoed these complexities when she described how it was a shame she had missed the Kalgoorlie show on her tour of *Chopped Liver*, and that she would have been "happy but sad" to be there because "I see a lot of my relations in jail that way and it'd be probably the only time I get to properly see them is when I take a show in there to them." When asked if her lived experience strengthened her ability to tackle the issues and do the work, Nazaree replied, "It definitely gives us an understanding of where those audience members and those community members are coming from, especially if you see that there's something that's been triggered in them and then they feel the need to unpack it." But she emphasised the need to take care of herself in these situations as well, "To make sure that I am actually unpacking that as a person myself." Nazaree also highlighted the need for performers to remain adaptable and not to "generalise" their own lived experiences to other communities: "Yes, you get the same characters everywhere you go, but every community is so unique, so you can never really say, 'Well, that worked great in Swan Hill, so of course it's going to work in Pukatja.'"

It was clear that interviewees found touring into prisons had the most impact in terms of cultural and psychological load. Melodie Reynolds-Diarra related a disturbing story about going into the protection unit of one of the prisons, where a convicted rapist had tried to intimidate her through body language and eye contact in a way that Melodie described as trying to "strip me back to the bone." She responded by standing up to him "energetically" during the introductions to the cast at the end of the show, holding eye contact, and shaking his hand strongly until he introduced himself. Of this incident, Melodie commented, "The story puts you in a place where you have to step up, shape up energetically, spiritually."

Performer Laila Thaker also related how touring for the first time into adult prisons with *Viral* had affected her, highlighting in a very real sense just how over-represented First Nations peoples are in the system.

> You realise all [these] other … things that you've got inside of you that you that you need to deal with, and I think that came to head when I did maybe the first or second show. … I was calculating how many fullas that we'd performed for at that point. … I can't even remember off the top of my head now, but it was a mass amount. I was just calculating, all of these men are in here, but they could be out with us. It was like, these men are just beautiful, caring, lovely, respectful, funny, genuine fullas and they're all in here and not out there with us in the community and it just made me really sad. I just remember feeling … really slack. I think that's when the penny drop happened for me. It's that reflecting of these mob are here and not with us in our community.

Melodie echoed this sentiment: "To see so many black faces [in prison] was kind of—statistically that was just a bit overwhelming in a way." For Laila, visiting the prison was confronting on another level as well, where she felt "racially vilified" by non-Indigenous staff:

> One thing I found confronting about the experience with *Viral*, probably - the going in and out of these prisons was pretty intense actually. Having to regularly deal with the really abrasive energies of the guards and the cops that were there was pretty hectic for me actually. … I'm just coming in as a performer, you know. Yeah, I just found that really confronting, each time.

Yet despite the emotional toll of entering these spaces, there remained a feeling that performers had a strong sense of responsibility to get on with the job and were equally gaining a great deal from the energy of their interactions with prison audiences. As *Chopped Liver* performer Isaac Drandic put it:

> I never felt too overloaded. I kind of always just knew that there's a job to do … And they [incarcerated audiences] didn't - that kind of heaviness wasn't transferred onto us anyway. Because they were so, they were full of light … they had light in their eyes. Like my cousin said, … they weren't there [in prison] for 50 minutes. … That's what kept us going for 150–200 shows. …That's what kept the energy up because they gave it to us. (Interview, 2021)

Similarly, Jesse Butler described how, although the prison environment was sometimes intimidating at first, he did not want to be sheltered from it and he always felt safe because he was among other Aboriginal or Torres Strait Islander people, and there was always someone to call upon in the Ilbijerri team for support if needed. Laila Thaker echoed these sentiments in describing the experience as "intense in a good way":

> Hearing the stories of, well not just Kamarra's experience but the experience of some of the fullas, the prisoners. … I found that pretty confronting as well. Then not only having to work with their stories but then you go meet them face-to-face, it just becomes that little bit more real. … So I obviously had to work through that. Kamarra was pretty good. I mean the whole process was really supportive. We always checked in on one another. We had all these really deadly cultural practices in place—meditation practices in place as well. I think that's what I love about working with Kamarra on this,

> not only because it's personal with her experience but also she's just like – I've never worked with someone like Kamarra as a director and a creator. She's just decolonising rehearsal spaces altogether. So while we were dealing with pretty intense themes and storytelling, it was all really – I felt safe. … I think that's probably the number one important thing of taking on a project like this, is that the foundations have to be strong and Kamarra and Ilbijerri made sure of that.

Laila's praise for Kamarra's methods points towards the need for consistency and ongoing training in attending to cultural safety, where in some cases there may have been different team members working in support roles who did not necessarily share the same skill level and rigorous approach to cultural safety as Kamarra.

The need to ensure cultural, emotional, and physical safety for performers was perhaps most evident in the experience of Shannon Hood, who joined the 2019 cast of *Viral* as an inexperienced performer who had recent lived experience of addiction and prison. While it had been extremely powerful to have someone in the cast whose experiences so closely mirrored those of the audience (as discussed later), this came with a stronger duty of care to ensure that Shannon could manage the pressures of learning the performance, getting up in front of an audience for the first time, and for some of those audience members to be closely connected to him. Shannon recalled how he had felt "overcome" at the beginning with the size of the role and the number of lines he had to learn in a short space of time. In addition to the pressure of performing, Shannon's portrayal of Merv brought up emotional connections and resonances that he was unable to set aside:

> Playing the old, broken sort of blackfulla who may have thought he'd wasted his life a bit and he had to build some bridges with his daughter before he passed away. Yeah, so there was that sort of emotional side going through it, which I know—you know of a lot of Elders that have passed away and you sort of think that they've probably passed away with a few regrets about life and the hand that they've been dealt. … I'm not going to say it was easy. (Interview, 2021)

Shannon was clear that he felt well supported by Kamarra and the other cast members throughout his time in *Viral*, but he went on to suffer a heart attack midway through the tour. Despite Shannon's belief that the heart attack was not necessarily a result of the performance and was "a long time coming," it provided a salutary lesson for Kamarra and the leadership team. While having someone like Shannon involved in the *Viral* was hugely beneficial on many levels, it is equally important to implement strong safety practices at all stages of a project.

Cultural Safety Processes and Practices

The examples cited above highlight the complexity and nuances of how lived experience and the colonial load affected different creative team members in different ways, with an acknowledgement that practices of self-care and care for each other were essential to managing such potentially charged work. The term "cultural safety," as introduced by Papps and Ramsden (1996) in the context of nursing and healthcare in New Zealand has gained traction in recent years in arts and education contexts, and the concept increasingly underpins many creative development, rehearsal, and touring practices in contemporary First Nations Theatre (Bracknell et al. 2021). The idea of creating "safe space" has long existed in social justice and by extension in community-engaged arts, with Bracknell et al. (2021, 384–385) building on the work of Arao and Clemens (2013) to articulate a "brave space" that could hold a creative workshop or rehearsal process that sometimes asked ensemble members to take risks or sit with discomfort—albeit within a framework for cultural, emotional, and physical safety. As discussed in Chap. 2, we also recognise that the content being explored through the health education works had to be tackled in a way that was both "safe and dangerous"—safely and authentically representing the issues, without shying away from the realities of, for example, confronting lived experiences and risky behaviours.

The benefit of strong cultural leadership in these projects meant that emotional safety, bravery, and sometimes danger could be balanced through a clear set of principles, protocols, and practices where creative teams with diverse lived experiences could thrive and do their best work. Kamarra has developed a strong framework for First Nations dramaturgy that holistically integrates responsibilities around cultural awareness, obligation, and representation when making works. This involves working in ways that are trauma informed and spiritually safe, which includes accounting for the diverse needs and manifestations of colonial load that artists may experience and working with an intentional awareness of the capacity for stories to both trigger and heal artists and audiences. Blayne Welsh (2018, 25) cites Shawn Wilson (2008) in describing how this occurred in the making of *Viral*, which promoted a sense of "relational accountability," "By using an exclusively Indigenous team, working via respectful collaborative practice and responsibly drawing from lived experiences and community voices." This included ritual aspects such as "sweeping" the space with gum leaves before commencing the process for the day (26) and holding space for all the different cultural backgrounds and experiences that are represented within a creative team or ensemble. Hyland, Syron, and Casey (2018, 6) reflect that rehearsal and performance spaces are not "neutral" or empty but "contain a legacy of theatre-making processes and practices that are also historically influenced by Western and European understandings of theatrical practice." They suggest artists use such methods to "counter the social, cultural and artistic traces of Western and European influences held within a rehearsal context" (7).

For the works described in this volume, these cultural elements and practices were woven to different degrees through every level of performance making from research and development through rehearsal to touring. A strong message from the interviews was the need to consistently support cultural, emotional, and even physical safety for creative teams and ensemble members through every stage. The potential for strong physical, emotional, and spiritual impacts of the performances on First Nations creative teams points to a need for safety, protection, and debriefing practices to underpin the works; and the research demonstrates that this has been achieved with varying degrees of success over the years. We suggest there can be an assumption that creatives can deal with these complex issues—particularly touring in prisons—which may not be the case in all instances. There is a need to not assume that the experience will be the same for everybody and to be responsive to different people's resilience, traumas, or triggers in developing plans for cultural safety within the works. Our interviews highlighted four ways in which performers were able to maintain a sense of cultural safety: a tight-knit and supportive team on tour and back at Ilbijerri; performers having strong self-care instincts and practices; strong cultural practices to open, close, and clear rehearsal and performance spaces; and formal and informal avenues for briefing and debriefing tours and individual performances.

As discussed in the previous section, several interviewees highlighted how their fellow performers and staff back at Ilbijerri were key in providing support during challenging times. In our yarn with Isaac Drandic, Kamarra pointed out how close the touring team had been for *Chopped Liver* at that time and that this may have contributed to Isaac's ability to not become "overloaded" and to just get on with the job. Isaac agreed that this was helpful in coping with the gruelling nature of touring:

> I suppose it was kind of about keeping the kind of energy up. It's a little bit like a long game … using a sports analogy or something. It would be a long-distance race or something that you just have to try and keep the energy up, keep your spirits up during the long tours like that.

Similarly, in discussion with Nazaree Dickerson, Kamarra pointed to the strength of the team on the *Scar Trees* tour, which helped to alleviate some of the potential risks of dealing with such traumatic material (family violence) with audiences who were victim-survivors:

> Thank God the team on *Scar Trees* was such a tightknit group and really had each other's backs. Because when we haven't had that on tours, it makes things a lot harder, and I just don't know how that show would have kind of been able to finish the tour if we didn't have such a strong team.

Testament to the strength of that team was their capacity to be responsive to the pressures of touring the show and share the load in terms of participating in the post-show yarning circle. Nazaree reflected,

> They've just finished a show, they're processing all those emotions as performers and then having to – there's that duty of care coming into community, knowing that … you might have someone revealing something extremely private and vulnerable about their own lives and you have to be emotionally available to deal with that, if you're asking them to sit in a yarning circle and reveal that information or even making the space open for that to happen.

She went on to explain that the cast created a "rotating roster" so that performers could sit out of the yarning circle and "have a breather" if needed.

Referring to his time in *Viral*, Shannon Hood talked about the importance of "camaraderie" and the need for the performance teams to "gee each other up." As an inexperienced performer, this was crucial to him gaining the confidence to go on stage. Nevertheless, due to different personalities and group dynamics, a strong, tight-knit team cannot be guaranteed, which potentially puts the emotional and cultural safety of all team members at risk. Facing such a situation on the 2018 *Viral* tour, Kamarra and Mary Quinsacara discussed the need for carefully managing such situations as they arise, as well as placing other mechanisms and safeguards in practice through every stage of a performance to hopefully prevent such situations from occurring in the first place.

As discussed in the previous section, Melodie Reynolds-Diarra highlighted the importance of strong self-care processes and practices in maintaining the safety and strength to deal with challenging environments such as prisons and to undertake such important work in communities. Nazaree Dickerson spoke about a specific occasion while touring *Scar Trees* where she had been deeply affected when a woman shared her personal story about being removed from a domestically violent situation. Nazaree felt that her prior experiences of touring with *Chopped Liver* and other shows in remote communities helped equip her with the necessary capacities for self-care and debriefing and that this included having informal debriefing yarns with other members of the touring party. But again, not all performers—especially those who are young or inexperienced—will have developed such skills and capacities as a matter of course. This suggests that future creative teams could benefit from training and development in self-care and the need for more formalised cultural safety practices, briefing, and debriefing surrounding the work.

In response to Melodie's experience in the men's prison, Kamarra acknowledged that although smoking and sweeping ceremonies were often performed at different stages of the tour, there was a need for "more extensive briefing and after care," particularly for women. This would take the form of mindful, spiritual, culturally based, empowering protective practice that is put in place when performers go in and that is cleared and held when they go out—a practice that is becoming more and more present in Kamarra's creative work. Mary Quinsacara felt that providing opportunities for yarning and debriefing for performers might have been a missing piece of the puzzle in the 2018 *Viral* tour, particularly in terms of performers having an opportunity to process the experience of going into prisons. There had been a process in place at the start, but it may have fallen away as the tour went on. For Mary, a non-Indigenous stage and tour manager, there was a lack of clarity around whose responsibility it was to instigate debriefing discussions with Mary understandably wishing not to step on any toes and to take her cues from the cast. Both Nazaree Dickerson and Jesse Butler spoke about how valuable it was to debrief informally with colleagues, but both acknowledged that having a formal structure was also valuable. Nazaree described her experience on *Scar*

Trees, where there were opportunities for a more organic process of yarning and debriefing, combined with a more formalised approach from the stage and production manager:

> She made sure that she asked everyone each day how are you doing today? Which I guess is generally part of a good workplace culture, but at the same time it's actually—there's a lot of—a lot more weight that comes with it when you're asking someone how they're doing after doing a show about someone that's experiencing domestic violence or Stolen Generation stuff. …So it's a bit—just tweaking and being more mindful. One thing that I've noticed is having to do that stuff in your own private time and it not actually being built into the schedule of a tour or a program, that's something that's always been missing from what I've seen in so many projects.

Jesse acknowledged that not everyone might feel able to just walk up to their colleagues and talk openly in this way and that a more formalised process at the end of each day might be helpful. Laila Thaker also spoke passionately about the value of debriefing to her during the 2018 *Viral* tour:

> I like debriefs. I'm all about the debriefs. I like to over analyse. I guess a lot of performers don't as well. So that's probably where there might have been tension. Somebody's debrief is just they want to debrief on their own, you know, just want to go home, have a cup of tea in their room or whatever, but I want to yarn about it.

While a formalised debriefing process might be demanding for some team members, the general feeling from the interviews was that to support the cultural safety of creative teams doing "heavy" work, there is a need for at least some kind of regular practice of debriefing that is negotiated amongst the team, and with a clear structure for who leads this process. Nazaree described this as a critical issue in terms of sustaining this crucial community practice:

> If that cultural care is not built into the program, you're having to do that yourself and it comes at a deficit near the end of the tour. You're worn out … burnt out. And that's not good, because then we can't continue to do the work.

Another critical element of this sustainability is the need not only to take care of creative teams but also to recognise the load that they carry with commensurate pay and conditions. As Laila Thaker observed, First

Nations artists like those at Ilbijerri are "overloaded" with demand for their work, and the cultural work of telling and holding community stories, although deeply rewarding, can carry with it extra responsibilities, obligations, and burdens. This must be recognised through the more practical and logistical elements of programming such as pay, benefits, tour scheduling, and the timely settlement of contracts.

Conclusion

This chapter has presented the health education performances as grounded in strong cultural leadership and underpinned by principles of cultural safety, collective responsibility, and relational accountability within all stages. These foundational aspects of the works essentially form the basis from which all other elements must spring. While there was some acknowledgement that safety practices and processes could be improved, this provided key learnings for subsequent projects like *The Score*, as will be discussed in the conclusion (Chap. 7). Also evident among our interviewees, however, was a deep respect for Kamarra and Ilbijerri's efforts in terms of providing a space in which creative teams' diverse lived experiences and positionalities could be valued and nurtured to support the work. First Nations ownership and leadership in projects such as these is also vital to the creative process and the capacity to integrate cultural elements respectfully and artfully within performances that speak to diverse Aboriginal and Torres Strait Islander communities' experiences. This is the focus of the next chapter, which presents findings around key aesthetic and performative elements of the shows that enabled them to artfully walk the line between "education" and "theatre" through the communication of a "gripping dramatic yarn."

References

Arao, Brian, and Kristi Clemens. 2013. From safe spaces to brave spaces. In *The Art of Effective Facilitation: Reflections From Social Justice Educators*, ed. Lisa M. Landreman, 135–150. Stylus Publishing LLC.

Bracknell, Clint, Kylie Bracknell, Susan Fenty Studham, and Luzita Fereday. 2021. Supporting the performance of Noongar language in *Hecate*. *Theatre, Dance and Performance Training* 12 (3): 377–395. https://doi.org/10.1080/19443927.2021.1943506.

Brodzinski, Emma. 2010. *Theatre in Health and Care*. Springer International Publishing.

Campbell, Alyson, and Dirk Gindt. 2018. Introduction. In *Viral Dramaturgies: HIV and AIDS in Performance in the Twenty-First Century*, ed. Alyson Campbell and Dirk Gindt, 343–365. Springer International Publishing.

Dudgeon, Pat, Abigail Bray, Dawn Darlaston-Jones, and Roz Walker 2020. Aboriginal Participatory Action Research: An Indigenous research methodology strengthening decolonisation and social and emotional wellbeing. Discussion Paper. Melbourne: The Lowitja Institute. https://www.lowitja.org.au/page/services/resources/Cultural-and-social-determinants/mental-health/aboriginal-participatory-action-research-an-indigenous-research-methodology-strengthening-decolonisation-and-social-and-emotional-wellbeing

Gee, Graham, Pat Dudgeon, Clinton Schultz, Amanda Hart, and Kerrie Kelly. 2014. Aboriginal and Torres Strait Islander social and emotional wellbeing. In *Working Together: Aboriginal and Torres Strait Islander Mental Health and Wellbeing Principles and Practice*, ed. Pat Dudgeon, Helen Milroy, and Roz Walker, 55–68. Canberra: Commonwealth of Australia.

Hyland, Nicola, Liza-Mare Syron, and Maryrose Casey. 2018. 'Turangawaewae': A Place to Stand in Contemporary Indigenous Performance in Australasia and Beyond. *Australasian Drama Studies 73*: 1–16. https://search.informit.org/doi/10.3316/informit.146442225934780

Keating, Clare. 2009. *'Chopped Liver' Evaluation Report*. Effective Change Pty Ltd. Melbourne: Ilbijerri Theatre Company. Supplied.

Laverack, Glenn, and Nastaran Keshavarz Mohammadi. 2011. What remains for the future: strengthening community actions to become an integral part of health promotion practice. *Health Promotion International* 26 (suppl_2): ii258–ii262. https://doi.org/10.1093/heapro/dar068.

Low, Katharine E. 2020. *Applied Theatre and Sexual Health Communication: Apertures of Possibility*. Palgrave Macmillan.

Papps, Elaine, and Irihapeti Ramsden. 1996. Cultural Safety in Nursing: The New Zealand Experience. *International Journal for Quality in Health Care* 8 (5): 491–497. https://doi.org/10.1093/intqhc/8.5.491.

Syron, Liza-Mare. 2021. *Rehearsal Practices of Indigenous Women Theatre Makers*. Springer International Publishing.

Verbunt, Ebony, Joanne Luke, Yin Paradies, Muriel Bamblett, Connie Salamone, Amanda Jones, and Margaret Kelaher. 2021. Cultural Determinants of Health for Aboriginal and Torres Strait Islander People–a Narrative Overview of Reviews. *International Journal for Equity in Health* 20: 1–9. https://link.springer.com/article/10.1186/s12939-021-01514-2.

Welsh, Blayne. 2018. The Hepatitis C Trilogy: A Case for Indigenous Theatre as a Contemporary Manifestation of Traditional Healing Business. *Australasian Drama Studies* 73: 20–41. https://search.informit.org/doi/abs/10.3316/ielapa.146479491877297.

Wilson, Shawn. 2008. *Research is Ceremony: Indigenous Research Methods*. Fernwood.

CHAPTER 5

The "Gripping Dramatic Yarn"

Abstract This chapter presents further findings from our study on the five health education works led by Kamarra Bell-Wykes and produced by Ilbijerri Theatre Company from 2006 to 2019. These findings draw on interviews conducted with eight practitioners who were involved over the years as performers, production staff, and advisors, a research yarn conducted between co-authors Sarah and Kamarra, and Kamarra's own critical reflections while putting together this volume. We also analysed documents and data from Ilbijerri's corporate archive and published works such as those by Clare Keating (*'Chopped Liver' Evaluation Report*. Effective Change Pty Ltd. Melbourne: Ilbijerri Theatre Company. Supplied,2009) and Blayne Welsh (The Hepatitis C Trilogy: A Case for Indigenous Theatre as a Contemporary Manifestation of Traditional Healing Business. *Australasian Drama Studies* 73: 20–41. https://search.informit.org/doi/abs/10.3316/ielapa.146479491877297, 2018). Utilising a quote from Isaac Drandic (one of the study's interview subjects), this chapter explores the second of three prominent themes within the data: the framing of the works as "gripping dramatic yarns" that centred cultural storytelling infused with authenticity, engaging characters, humour, and strong acting and performance skills. As we explore in Chap. 6, these elements enabled the works to deftly walk the line between entertainment and education, effectively promoting audience engagement and connection and supporting the health education and messaging. As such, we continue to argue that the works progress the dramaturgies of

S. Woodland, K. Bell-Wykes, *First Nations Australian Theatre for Health Equity*, https://doi.org/10.1007/978-3-031-65506-7_5

wellbeing, strength, and resistance that characterise contemporary First Nations theatre in Australia.

Keywords First Nations theatre • Theatre in education • Applied theatre • Arts and health • Theatre for health education

In his 2021 interview for this study, Isaac Drandic, an original cast member from *Chopped Liver* and acclaimed theatre maker in his own right, described the work as "a gripping dramatic yarn." His comment was made in the context of a discussion about why the work was so successful in engaging audiences and enabling them to talk safely and openly about hepatitis C. While scholar Emma Brodzinski (2010) notes longstanding criticisms of theatre for health education as being message focused over and above artistic considerations, the works discussed in this volume have been carefully crafted to walk a convincing line between education and gripping theatre. Although some performances were more successful than others at doing so, as will be discussed further below, it was achieved through a combination of strong cultural metaphors that supported the health messaging; compelling, authentic storylines that reflected the audience's experiences; engaging and nuanced characters; the inclusion of humour and comedy; and sophisticated performance aesthetics that included high levels of acting and performance skills. In essence, this supports the cultural framing of the works as 'yarns' both as true-to-life stories told in elegantly simple, entertaining ways for the purpose of transmitting important cultural messages and as vehicles for creating safe spaces for open talk or yarning about the health issues being explored.

Cultural Framing Through Storytelling

> Kamarra: When you're sitting around a fire at night … it can become a little bit competitive. You know, who has the best yarn? So, we're really entertaining each other. … We're all historians. We're storytellers very innately, and so I think … we've got a lot of good storytellers and we've got a lot of funny storytellers. … So, we really, we put some effort in to how we set it up and how that timing comes in … there's a kind of standard, I think, that comes from the community. (Interview, 2021)

Melodie Reynolds-Diarra reflected on how a good story "can be told anywhere with just the bare essentials or just the voice" (interview, 2021). Isaac Drandic discussed how this was vital for *Chopped Liver,* which needed to be toured economically in terms of set and production equipment: "The story has to be interesting because you've got nothing [else] to fall back on." Nazaree Dickerson pointed out how this minimalism was part of the "magic" in productions, where their "scaled back" simplicity was integral to the yarn. She recalled audience members "getting a kick" out of a scene in *Chopped Liver* where a baby was represented by just a blanket wrapped up.

> That's what … so many of our cultures hold is that storytelling and playfulness that comes so naturally … so the fact that you get to do this in contemporary theatre is what I love and then showing Mob how easy it is. Because any blackfulla can tell you they see their family members do this all the time, tell a yarn. There's always somebody that can tell a yarn really playfully and use something, a mundane object, like a remote, to be a phone or things like that. That's what I loved about it. (Interview, 2021)

In approaching the writing, Kamarra has always been clear that finding a compelling story first was critical and that the health messaging would then follow. For her, this entailed making the right choices around character, world, and truth and finding the emotional arc of the story. *Chopped Liver* and *Viral – Are You the Cure?* were successful in this regard because they depicted multiple perspectives on the issue through a range of characters. This ensured that the hepatitis C virus was represented not just through a single story but through an intergenerational relationship where different stories came together. Kamarra sees this as vital to representing a diversity of community experiences and taking care not to represent First Nations peoples or at-risk groups as homogenous. Within this, Kamarra experimented with different styles of theatre and performance so that the work could capture different yarning styles in approaching audiences. Works such as *Body Armour* and *North West of Nowhere* were not quite as successful in this regard, due in part to the fact that there had been some interference from a reference group member, who wanted specific health facts and messaging to be inserted into the scripts. This heavy-handed approach to messaging, discussed in more detail in Chap. 6, could be seen to compromise the artistic integrity within the works that reflects some of the criticism levelled at theatre for health education mentioned above.

Extending on this, Melodie Reynolds-Diarra spoke at length about the legacy of colonisation that has led to First Nations peoples regarding health information and statistics with fear and suspicion because they are usually delivered by non-Indigenous people in "oppressing" ways. From her perspective, the framing of such information through a "playful" and engaging dramatic yarn helped audiences, particularly in prisons, to lower their guard and connect with a more child-like curiosity:

> In that moment there you get the information through, you get them remembering and [feeling the] emotion and what happened in that scene, [as] opposed to the statistics. … I keep on coming back to the word, 'visceral' because I suppose it's harder to tune off from someone standing in front of you telling a story. … It opens up all that thing to that child within; you know, 'Let me sit down now, [be patient], let me tell you this yarn, and throughout this yarn, it's about these two people here. This is what they went through.' … That's not pushing anything onto anyone … it leaves it open.

This points to the strength of these works in terms of their primary purpose—to impart important health information—which will be discussed further in the next chapter. However, it also highlights the need for such information to be delivered in an aesthetically engaging, culturally safe, culturally relevant way, that is, through entertaining yarning. In a sense, it decolonises health promotion and education so that audiences feel empowered, rather than oppressed, by a meaningful exchange of information through storytelling.

Findings from the data show that a key strength of the five health education works was their cultural framing, which included engaging storytelling as discussed above, as well as potent cultural metaphors, imagery, and reference points from both contemporary First Nations cultural experience and more traditional elements of history, ceremony, and spirituality. These will be unpacked in more detail in the sections that follow; however, they are undoubtedly key to the levels of engagement from audiences and the capacity for the performances to deliver health messaging and education effectively. As Blayne Welsh (2018, 39) pointed out in relation to *Viral*,

> In the making of *Viral*, the director Kamarra Bell-Wykes employed historical Indigenous performance practices—such as the use of humour, dance and story—to communicate a particular trauma (sorry business) associated

> with living with hepatitis C. In presenting [it] through a cultural framework, the performance spoke directly to the issues and allowed knowledge transfer in a way much like we have done for thousands of years.

Peter Waples-Crowe highlighted the importance of having "an intertwined cultural story" in the works and how this was a signature of Kamarra's work, "It might be—not a Dreamtime story—but a story from Country that relates to it," giving the example of the brolga that featured in *North West of Nowhere* (interview, 2021). The striking presence of the tree in the set for *Scar Trees* embodied the narrative's cultural metaphor foregrounding the resilience and strength of scar trees (Fig. 2.5).

> Kirra: Cos at first it's like they're not even there, the scars. Nobody knows unless you look. Then you first see 'em and it's kinda ugly, like it looks like the tree is in pain or broken or whatever. But then when you look closer, it's like: actually it's beautiful. Cos it shows the past. Shows that we were here. And how we lived. And that we existed. And what we went through. What the tree went through. And it's alive still. You know? And if you frame it right and hold it in the right light, it is beautiful. (*Scar Tree*, 2019)

Perhaps one of the most arresting examples of an integration between traditional and contemporary cultural elements occurred in *Viral*, where the creative team developed a dance demonstrating the connection between intravenous sharing practices, ceremonial rituals, cultural substitution, and the impact of colonial disease. Starting in traditional form, the performers prepared and applied ochre together before dancing in harmony with Spirit around the fire. The 'traditional' rhythm was then interrupted by a banjo as the dance repeated and mutated to demonstrate the crushing, mixing, and sharing of a 'dirty hit'. Finally, the 'virus' infected their bodies and the performers heaved and convulsed, eventually collapsing on the ground. Welsh (2018) describes how this dance was used in *Viral* to depict the contemporary rituals of drug use as being a colonising "replacement" for traditional cultural rituals (Fig. 5.1). This moves the work beyond simply depicting risky or harmful behaviours and towards a deeper understanding of the structural inequities that have led to such impacts on communities. Kamarra's goal was to create a moment that spoke to the message as well as the deeper spiritual truths within First Nations cultures, and she was surprised at the effect it had on audiences.

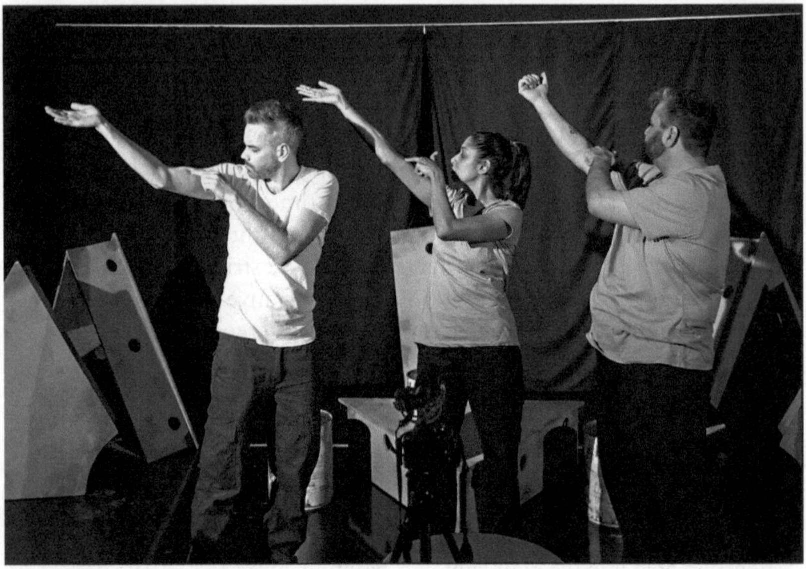

Fig. 5.1 (L-R) Jesse Butler, Laila Thaker, and Blayne Welsh, *Viral – Are You the Cure?* Image by Tiffany Garvie (2018)

Audience feedback from the 2018 tour indicated that this scene had a powerful impact:

> The scene where they shot up to the sound of the Indigenous rhythm sticks really blew me away and was such a powerful image.
>
> A very powerful performance by all. I will be haunted by the scene where cultural ritual evolves in to shooting up ritual. (Audience survey responses, *Viral* 2018)

However, the prison audiences surprisingly cracked up laughing at the dance and explained later, "You can't do that in here! We can't believe you did that!" with a joy that spoke to the dramatic freedom theatre can create inside the highly restricted context behind prison walls.

Jesse Butler described how important it was to include these kinds of performative elements but also how crucial it was for First Nations audiences to see themselves and their stories represented on stage:

> Understanding what's going to work and bringing Indigenous performance styles into what we're doing also makes Mob feel a part of it. They feel like they recognise not just the words but also some of the things that are going on on stage, these little performances, and these rituals that we were involving in the show was something that they do as well. So, it wasn't just a theatre show. It was like we're doing what we do in life, and we're doing it on stage. (Interview, 2020)

This points towards the critical element of authenticity that will be discussed further below. By integrating strong cultural metaphors with contemporary issues, audiences were able to relate deeply to what they were seeing. As one teacher noted of *North West of Nowhere*, "The performance was fabulous. I loved the cultural content and the contemporary nature of the dialogue. I am sure it benefitted our students in a range of ways" (Ilbijerri Theatre Company 2014, 6). Other elements, such as the style of storytelling and humour, were also critical in creating this kind of connection, as will be discussed further below.

Nevertheless, Kamarra and Isaac Drandic discussed how integrating cultural references and content could have challenges in terms of touring through diverse First Nations communities across the country. Isaac recalled touring in Kalgoorlie, where he had some cousins:

> Their first language is Wangkatha, or Pitjantjatjara, or one of the desert languages out there, there would have been a kind of language disconnect. There would have been a cultural disconnect. Talking about Expo '88, they don't know what Expo '88 is. Yeah, I do remember that actually. I do remember that it wasn't the usual response that we got from pretty much 90 per cent of the other communities and prisons that we went to. Yeah, there was a huge kind of cultural gap there between us.

This was part of the reason why Kamarra was keen to develop a more community-responsive model such as that found in *The Score*, which would allow space for more diverse languages and cultural stories.

In terms of cross-cultural readings of the works, responses from non-Indigenous audiences in the surveys were positive, and several creatives interviewed for the research indicated that the themes and storylines being covered might be accessible to a non-Indigenous audience. Melodie Reynolds-Diarra suggested that non-Indigenous audiences who were "open enough" and "without prejudice" would "be drawn along" to see the plays. Speaking about *Chopped Liver*, Isaac Drandic pointed out,

> There's enough kind of stuff in there, relationship stuff and metaphors around wanting to be a big shot. The little skimp wanted to be a goanna and there's enough connections in there that, yeah, connect to non-Indigenous folk as well, for sure.

On the other hand, there was a sense that the performances would connect more strongly for a First Nations audience, given that, as Jesse Butler pointed out, the plays were "written mostly for Mob." Melodie observed that in some spaces such as prisons, there could be a more "immersive" relationship between First Nations and non-Indigenous people, resulting in a shared understanding of jokes and other references but that the strength of cultural references sometimes resulted in a satisfying power shift:

> So, they got our jokes, they already got our humour but sometimes … there's a moment where you see a power dynamic in an audience where the blackfullas are, 'This shit—this is *our* song.' So that they're appreciating it in a different way to the non-Indigenous people that are in the audience, and it just actually creates a bit of a power dynamic; like, 'This one's for us,' you know? And it's just nice to see that shape—that power kind of shift sometimes in those spaces because it's generally the other way around.

This points towards a critical quality of the performances as being empowering for First Nations audiences, which is discussed further in Chap. 6.

Performances of *Viral* to largely non-Indigenous school students were not as successful. Kamarra observed, "You could see they wanted to connect, but it was like, this is not your lived experience. …I don't think they kind of knew what to take away from it as well, though they tried really hard" Jesse agreed with this assessment:

> I think with the Indigenous kids we've got that connection straightaway. … Maybe they've had a relative in some situations, whereas even an Indigenous person who hasn't been through anything like that has Mob. … Every Indigenous kid knows an alcoholic, or a drug addict, or someone who's been thrown in jail, or someone who's been racially vilified—something. There's always something to connect with.

Jesse went on to discuss his experience of performing to non-Indigenous health workers: "We'd be in some health centre with all white health workers. The show is just going over their heads and they were like - and you're kind of like, 'That was hard.'" Later, he also discussed how potentially disempowering for First Nations audience members it could be to have non-Indigenous people in the yarning circle afterwards sharing their own stories and experiences in detail: "That's great but we're not here for that right now. Read the room." Kamarra has always been adamant that the primary audience for these health education performances is First Nations peoples, despite there being occasions on some tours when the work has not necessarily reached that audience to the optimal degree.

The evidence above supports the framing of the health education works as "gripping dramatic yarns" with cultural storytelling at their heart, deliberately aimed at First Nations audiences, and explicitly dealing, not only with the complexities of the health issues themselves but also with the wider structural inequities that have disadvantaged Australia's first peoples since colonisation. We now dig more deeply into four specific features that supported these gripping yarns as highlighted most prominently within the data: authenticity, humour, characters, and strong acting and performance skills.

Authenticity

The element of authenticity within the health education works might seem somewhat artificially separated from other elements that contributed to their effectiveness as "gripping yarns." It was no doubt a combination of cultural elements, storylines, characters, dialogue, and emotional content of the productions that felt authentic or true to life for audience members. Nevertheless, this was a theme that repeatedly came up in our research and is a signature of the way Kamarra approaches this kind of work. For her, writing *Chopped Liver* was a deeply personal project, given that she was, at the time, living with hepatitis C.

> I guess the thing that was a little bit strange about the whole process was—and I don't know whether the person that approached me as the writer knew this or not—but I was living with hepatitis C, and I hadn't told anybody about that. [And] despite that, I still didn't actually know that much about the virus, although I knew a lot about the shame, and I knew a lot about the emotional truth, and I guess that was the thing that really made a big difference.

Kamarra's commitment to finding the emotional truth within the works has remained in place ever since, with a strong conviction that this is the only way for these kinds of works to resonate on a personal and cultural level for audiences so that they can then swallow the "medicine" of health education and messaging.

This was also reflected elsewhere in the data. As Jesse Butler observed of the *Viral* workshops and performances in prisons, "It's *their* story. That's why it has such an impact." Blayne Welsh (2018, 32) describes in his paper, "In referring to how similar some of the character's … experiences were to his own, one inmate asked, 'Have you been to my house?'" Isaac Drandic described how the story and dialogue in *Chopped Liver* were "very identifiable to people."

> We were speaking the language that they speak. It wasn't 'Home and Away' language, it wasn't upper end kind of language, it wasn't Shakespeare or anything like that. It was plain talk. We sounded like the people that we were taking the show to.

Written audience feedback in both the post-show surveys and the guestbook for *Viral* contained numerous references to the truth of the performance:

> Fantastic. Beautiful and emotional and real. Thank you.
> Realistic, triggering, emotional, raw, brilliant.
> The show was amazing. The emotion that was experienced was truly real. Well done.
> Very powerful. Had me feeling it was real and not acting.
> Great performance, great acting, really engaging. I love the realness. Thank you for spreading the word and encouraging healing in the community.
> Fantastic and very creative production. Very realistic scenarios.
> I was very moved by this play. I liked the honesty even though it was very confronting.

The quotes above illustrate how important the emotional intensity and authenticity of the story were in enabling audiences to sit with some of the confronting aspects of the performance. As cited in the previous section, Melodie Reynolds-Diarra explains how this emotional truth is key to communicating the deeper complexities of the issue behind the health facts and statistics. Peter Waples-Crowe echoed this sentiment, describing how important it was to integrate the messaging with an "honest" story:

> The plays dealt with issues that are often supressed, or not talked about, or so stigmatised, and they did it in a really realistic, honest way, upfront and… I think a lot of people know messages, but when they're intertwined into people's lives, then it can make a really big difference.

Jesse Butler had much to say about the authenticity of the stories and performances and seemed to connect with this idea deeply as an actor. For him, it was extremely intimidating yet satisfying to interpret the role of Kev/Doc in *Viral* in front of a prison audience:

> Kamarra is an incredible director and very authentic herself. So, she really wants that in the performance. That was kind of drilled into us, how real we had to be and it was such an incredible acting experience it made me a better actor to be in those situations.

He went on to discuss how the authenticity of the story and its telling were connected directly to the cultural practice of yarning:

> That's what authenticity is all about, it's just about being real in that place and not trying to do this show. You're not trying to… perform in front of them. You're just telling a story. You're having a yarn. That's the beauty of performing in front of Mob as well because I think they—Mob understand performance.

Melodie Reynolds-Diarra discussed how important authenticity was for the *Chopped Liver* performances to hold the attention of audiences in prisons, where few people would be used to watching live performance, while at the same time delivering a health message that might otherwise be stigmatising. For her, it was Kamarra's "non-judgemental" and "engaging writing" that enabled the works to overcome these hurdles:

> [The] writing grabbed people because it was at their vibrational level, their lingo, their recognition in historical events that were placing them in the moment. It was an honest story of two people that they could relate to but it's not pointing fingers at them. …As soon as you have the non-judgemental stuff coming through, you've got an opening for it to be healed in a way of the inmates and people like - feel like it's easier to talk to someone about it because they've just seen it live and it's not removed on television or a screen as such. It's someone viscerally feeling and saying those words and those emotions and getting through their problems.

Here, Melodie not only describes the authenticity of the performances but also their "visceral" power as live events, opening a space for connection and discussion.

An additional element of authenticity in *Viral's* second tour was the presence of Shannon Hood in the role of Merv, whose own life experiences mirrored those of many audience members and whose role as a recognisable community member with no previous performance experience had impact and currency. Jesse Butler reflected on this:

> There were a lot of comments from other people [about] how much they appreciated him … because he had been through so much himself and I think he knew a lot of people we were actually performing to and … the thing that really struck me was how it was so real, and it was about more than a performance.

Shannon's presence in the show added a layer of engagement for audience members who could see themselves, not only in his character but also in the man himself and his story. This had wider implications for both Shannon and his audiences that will be discussed further later, but certainly the presence of a person on stage with lived experience of the issues under investigation contributed to the authenticity of the piece. It was Shannon's presence in the performance as an untrained actor with lived experience that in part informed Kamarra's decision to adopt the participatory model for her most recent work *The Score,* where community members would be inducted into performances, thereby increasing potential connections and engagement for community audiences.

We discuss specific elements such as character, humour, and performance skills below; however, it is important to note that the sense of authenticity within these performances contributes on a broader scale to the project of decolonising both theatre and health education or promotion. As Maryrose Casey (2012) suggests, notions of authenticity in contemporary First Nations theatre have often been dictated by the colonising powers, who have historically set the parameters and expectations for what are considered authentic representations of "Aboriginality" on Australian stages, creating an "economy of authenticity." Paola Balla (2017) similarly discusses how White people's expectations are "tied up in authentic ideas about Aboriginality itself. It correlates with the idea[s] about traditional art and traditional people, and us being urban, so therefore…not real" (as cited in Thorner et al. 2018, 279). Works such as the ones we discuss here, led by First Nations creatives and made for First Nations audiences, therefore assert sovereignty over the stage, foregrounding the authentic stories and nuanced identities of contemporary Aboriginal and Torres Strait Islander peoples and (in this case) their authentic experiences of structural health and wellbeing inequities in settler colonial Australia.

Engaging and Nuanced Characters

A key aspect of creating a sense of authenticity in these works was to incorporate heightened yet familiar characters whom audience members felt they could recognise from their own communities. The lead characters in *Chopped Liver* are "Uncle" and "Aunty" archetypes Jim and Lynn, a likable couple haunted by their high-risk pasts and seeking a better future. These characters appealed to a broad First Nations audience regardless of their experience with hep C and were great vehicles to explore the associated stigma, shame, and daily survival associated with the virus.

> Jim: Deep down I love her more than life itself but this hep C thing's floored me. Like someone's punched me in the gut and I can't get my breath back. Can't unsay what I've said. Can't!
>
> Lynne: Can't look me in the eye. Deep down I know he doesn't mean it. He wants the baby more than I do but can't talk things through… Says forget it—we'll forge on. I think if he can forget it, maybe I can. (Bell-Wykes 2018a, 29)

For *Body Armour*, which addresses hep C transmission among adolescents, the characters needed to demonstrate the various societal and cultural intersections of the issue while creating an engaging performance for young people.

For *Viral*, the artistic team—informed by the community workshops—created three characters who were at different stages of the virus. This was essential in representing the diversity of the community and the different reasons people were not taking up the available treatment. Some of the audience feedback for *Viral* identified the characters specifically as being integral to the success of the play:

> The characters were really well developed and their complexities showed so well.
> It was fantastic. Very complex, powerful, and thought provoking. It dealt with the characters in a respectful and compassionate manner.
> The play was great and I think theatre is great educational tool and people can identify with the characters. (*Viral* 2018, audience survey)

Shannon Hood reflected on the challenge of playing dual characters in *Viral*, Lewis, one of the white documentarians, and Merv, the older protagonist who had contracted hepatitis C. Shannon joined the cast, completely new to acting, and drew on his own lived experiences to play Merv:

> I felt like I had a bit of Merv in me anyway. It was just about trying to adapt that to a character that the people in the audience could relate to. Whether it be their uncle, their father, their brother, something like that. But I think everyone out in the community has a Merv in their life so it was just about putting Merv across in a sense that, Merv was bitter and angry, but also Merv was sorrowful and remorseful about his relationship with his daughter. It was just trying to get that balance in between. (Interview, 2021)

Shannon then spoke about how important it was to give nuance to the character, not only for the integrity of the show but also for his own emotional wellbeing in performing the role:

> I didn't want to make Merv to be an angry, old black man that just hated the world. I wanted Merv to come across how I felt when I got over my addictions and all of the things that I thought about when I was going through that. I just tried to sprinkle a little bit of that on top and that also made me feel a little bit comfortable and not be triggered or anything like that with any previous problems that I had.

As discussed earlier, Shannon's portrayal of Merv, particularly in the prison shows, contributed to the authenticity of the work and strengthened the messaging by presenting a peer with lived experience who could therefore be seen as a role model to audiences.

Shannon's instincts to go for nuance in his portrayal of Merv highlight another important factor in the success of these works. In all the works, Kamarra was committed to portraying a cross-spectrum of characters. This may include stereotypes—as there are truths to stereotypes and they can serve a purpose—but a range of other more nuanced characters who make different choices was included as well. There was also care taken around representation, where, for example, in the portrayal of the Nella in *North West of Nowhere*, who is 'slut-shamed' by her peer group claims back her power over her sexuality and identity by challenging the toxic assumptions commonly projected onto young women. Another strength of the works is the representation of First Nations communities in all their own diversity, including avoiding heteronormativity. As health worker Peter Waples-Crowe observed, "I was always uplifted to see that there were queer characters in the plays as well." Writing about theatre-based HIV prevention programs in the Asia Pacific region, Helen Cahill (2017) cautions against goodie/baddie tropes, suggesting that these can often reactivate stigmatising constructs that connect morality to disease. She highlights how focusing on relations between characters can assist in exploring how cultural codes and expectations often dictate behaviour, and this is an approach that has typically been adopted for these works. There is also a sense that the characters must serve the action and authenticity of the story and the relationships within it, rather than be shoe-horned into the performance as didactic vehicles for health messaging—as can often be the case in educational theatre. Even in *North West of Nowhere*, where Kamarra felt some pressure to include a health worker character to convey some of the key health information, she developed this character into an old man shapeshifter—a recognisable cultural archetype—in an effort to retain some of the authenticity and integrity of the play.

As in many educational plays, the 'hero' or protagonist in *North West of Nowhere*—Wyatt—was portrayed as someone with a choice to make, who was not endowed with risky behaviours but was rather in the stage of contemplating doing things differently. The risky behaviours were represented by an older antagonist, still likeable and recognisable to the community. Cuz, another recognisable cultural archetype, reflects the idea that everybody has an older bad-influencing cousin or relative who acts like a clown and should know better but does not. This allowed young audiences to witness an older person behave stupidly and presented an opportunity to exercise better judgment. Even though Wyatt is being teased for not being 'cool', he has an opportunity to make the harder choice. This approach echoes educational theatre works that are influenced by Theatre of the Oppressed (Boal 1985), offering the audience a protagonist in whom they can invest, supporting them to make healthy choices, while potentially being influenced by an antagonist, in this case Cuz. The two older characters (Cuz and Ol' Man) also represent the intergenerational scope of health and wellbeing in communities, which is also reflected in *Chopped Liver*, *Viral*, and *Scar Trees*. This demonstrates how knowledge is transmitted in Aboriginal and Torres Strait Islander cultures, also creating access points for diverse community audiences and situating the responsibility for community wellbeing with the whole community rather than centring the behaviour of specific individuals.

Humour

A vital aspect of the "gripping dramatic yarn" from a cultural perspective is humour, which was consistently deployed to great effect throughout the health education works discussed here. Humour not only provided a counterpoint to the seriousness of the issues being discussed but also gave depth and dimension to the characters and stories. It was also used as a vehicle for mocking the colonial systems surrounding health and wellbeing for First Nations audiences, as in the case of the non-Indigenous documentary filmmakers in *Viral*, who embodied the patronising, ill-informed, inappropriate behaviours of White "do-gooders" (Welsh 2018, 28). In *Viral*, the cameo roles of caricature prison guards Shaz and Daz brought comic relief while expressing the systematic failures of the prison system, proving to be an audience favourite particularly amongst incarcerated audiences.

Shaz: It's a cesspool.
Daz: I call it the 'Core'.
Shaz: Where molten lava of shit goes down on a daily basis.
Lewis: Can I ask about the drugs that get through here?
Shaz: No comment.
Daz: I do not know what you are talking about. (Viral - Are you the Cure? 2018)

The inclusion of humour was critical to winning over audiences in prison, where Kamarra was aware that performances would need to be especially engaging to break down suspicion and avoid being seen as "naff." The drug mixing and injecting dance in *Viral* described earlier provided the kind of shock value for prison audiences associated with dark comedy, eliciting strong reactions and laughter at the audacity of showing this in front of prison officers in a highly restricted environment.

To engage its young audiences, in *North West of Nowhere,* Kamarra decided to ridiculously signpost the "insert health information here" with an absurd but very real comical prop—a box of plastic "cocks" concealed as shiny bright bananas, much to the despair and delight of the audience.

> Old man: Those are the latest model. Very realistic. Somehow people feel more comfortable when they're wrapped up in something –still cant get 'em to use a bloody condom though – go figure. (Bell-Wykes 2018b, 36)

This somewhat clunky but playful action became the show's highlight and served to mock the theatre in education form itself and good-naturedly undercut the idea of 'serious' messaging (Fig. 5.2).

Helen Cahill (2017) notes that humour can give permission to participants to engage freely with explicit sexual content and taboo topics. Humour provides an opening for people to relax, let down their guard, and feel more able to connect with the story and the performers on stage. It is therefore a critical aspect of reducing the stigma associated with challenging topics such as addiction and sexual health. As one teacher pointed out after a performance of *Body Armour* at their school, "What a fantastic performance. Students laughed and learned - a great combination"

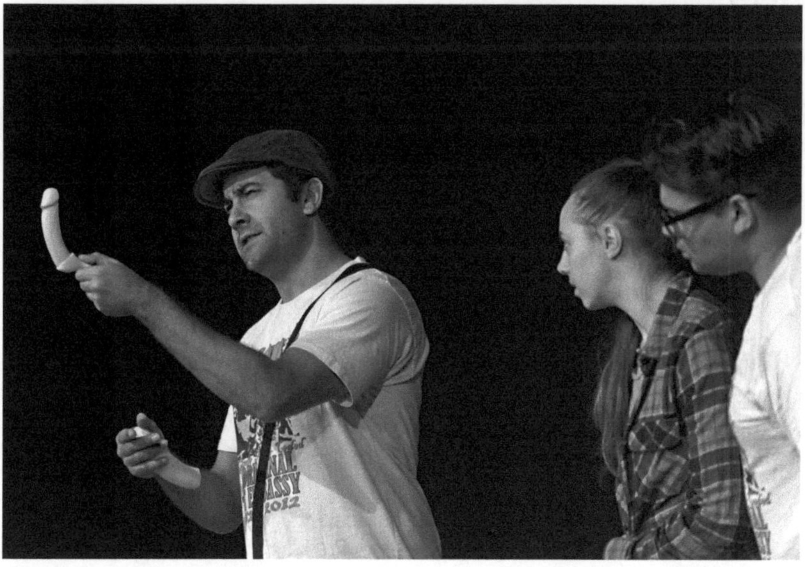

Fig. 5.2 (L-R) James Henry, Carly Sheppard, and Ian Michael, *North West of Nowhere*. Image by Brent Edwards (2015)

(Ilbijerri Theatre Company 2013, 5). Kamarra's tenet (under John Romeril's wise advice) to "Get 'em laughing then punch 'em in the guts!" (see Chap. 2) was particularly relevant to the first energetic and comedic scenes of *Chopped Liver*, which worked to "win the audience over" before any mention of hepatitis C. Audience reflections from the first tour highlighted this vital combination of drama and humour:

> The play has dignity and power. It is so 'un-pious.' To turn sadness into humour is a great achievement.
> How well the play is written – its ability to deal so seamlessly with so many complex issues about health and life and relationships, with both drama and humour.
> Yeah, deadly as. Great way to inform people. Funny side of a disease that has a big impact on a lot of people. Good to let people know to get over the shame job and get checked out and learn how to live with it.
> Transforming 'heavy duty messages' about hepatitis C through the humour and humanity of the play, which in turn ensures that the messages are actually received and recalled.
> (Keating 2009, 6–17)

In a recent literature review of "humour-based strategies" in 13 global public health studies (Miller et al. 2021, 568), humour was identified as a "useful tool for increasing awareness and help-seeking behaviour for public health priorities, particularly those associated with stigma." In addition, there is a strong cultural tradition of using humour in performance, particularly to provide a counterpoint to serious or traumatic material. As Kamarra pointed out,

> When you're writing a play about something that's really heavy, it's like you've got to go even harder the other way to find the humour and the light. ...And particularly because it's such a language of blackfullas, that humour, cracking humour is essential.

Blayne Welsh (2018, 36–37) also describes the crucial role of humour in First Nations storytelling in relation to *Viral*:

> Just as our ancestors have done for thousands of years, in *Viral*, community and inmate audiences were given permission to laugh at the everyday trauma of living with hepatitis C, and being incarcerated, providing the opportunity to potentially make some light of their immediate realities.

As discussed in Chap. 3, Maryrose Casey (2013) notes that many of the monodramas in her study used humour to undercut trauma and the painful experiences of racial prejudice. Jacob Boehme's *Blood on the Dancefloor* provided a unique lens on the issue of HIV by incorporating irreverent "black humour" (Campbell and Graffam 2018, 352). Incorporating humour is therefore much more than just a way to engage audiences and pull them into the health messaging. As First Nations scholar Angeline Hurley (2015) states, "Considering the impact of colonisation, racism, conflict and oppression, the health and wellbeing of Aboriginal and Torres Strait Islander peoples prevails through humour."

Strong Acting and Performance Skills

The strength of the acting and performance skills demonstrated by cast members since *Chopped Liver* premiered in 2006 is another element identified throughout our research as being critical to the success of the health education works. While applied or educational theatre's artistic value is often criticised in comparison to mainstream or mainstage productions, Kamarra has always maintained a sense of determination that high production values, acting, and performance skills must not be compromised in these works. Audience feedback for *Viral* highlighted how important this element was in conveying the story and messaging:

> So powerfully, very moving. The acting was wonderful. Thank you.
> I really enjoyed this play. Honestly think yous [sic] are very good actors and should continue your plays.
> The actors drew us in and had us there the whole time which is the best thing you can to so well done to all of yous [sic].
> Great performance, great acting, really engaging. I love the realness. Thank you for spreading the word and encouraging healing in the community.
> I thought the acting and overall performance was superb.
> Fantastic performance and strong ensemble work.
> Amazing performances. Each actor was beautifully connected and committed throughout the whole performance! Brilliant work. (*Viral* 2018/2019, audience guest books and surveys)

This supports Peter Waples-Crowe's assertion cited earlier that the performances provided an example of "Aboriginal excellence" that would reinforce a sense of empowerment and positive identity among audiences, as discussed further in Chap. 6.

In casting these performances, Ilbijerri has always recognised the need for actors to be both captivating in performance and grounded in their ability to connect with community members in an intimate, non-theatre space. While in theatre in education actor-teachers are traditionally known to draw together skills in performance, pedagogy, and audience engagement (Cooper 2013), we argue that there is a deeper cultural practice at play in these works. As Melodie Reynolds-Diarra pointed out, the performances open a collective space for healing, which endows the performers with a sense of relational responsibility (Wilson 2008): "You give this story and then it's like they give their stories back. …So, in that, there's almost like an alchemy that kind of happens, as an exchange that happens." Melodie went on to say that this required performers, particularly in spaces such as prisons, to be open-hearted and non-judgemental.

The idea of performers in these works building relational skills and "giving back" to communities is also discussed in more detail in Chap. 6; however, several of the actors involved discussed how the nature of the work built their skills as performers. The health education works produced by Ilbijerri have been a strong training ground for First Nations actors who have gone onto mainstage theatre, film, and television. Melodie Reynolds-Diarra observed,

> I suppose as an actor it was one of the biggest … challenge[s] in honing your skills and, for a start, doing a two hander because anything with a small amount of actors or a solo is pretty daunting because you're holding the energy for that long of a show in general.

Melodie went on to describe how particularly challenging this was when also trying to deliver a health message at the same time but that the simplicity of *Chopped Liver,* as described earlier by Nazaree Dickerson, enabled her to develop strong skills in communicating the story: "As an actor, that's a beautiful challenge to work with and to use your craft is playing the different facets of this story and going wholeheartedly into them as well."

As discussed above, Jesse Butler talked about how the authenticity of the performances and the challenge of delivering a convincing performance inside a prison helped hone his acting skills. *Viral* tour manager Mary Quinsacara supported this in her recollections: "What I observed with Jesse is how when we were in those particular spaces it's like he had to put on a top, top fucking performance to sell it" (interview, 2020).

Jesse described his personal journey of developing these skills in a community context:

> The places you're performing in, sometimes kitchens, libraries, just a room between another room, yeah, which at first I guess is pretty intimidating. … You look out into the audience while you're performing and you're seeing … people who are in these situations that you're actually trying to tell a story about instead of just a theatre audience. So, yeah just I guess the shock to begin with, but then also that finding comfortability in performing in a community centre.

Jesse's journey highlights the important skill of "selling" the characters to a community audience who are experts in the lived experiences being portrayed on stage. Isaac Drandic pointed out that there needed to be an instant sense of trust or rapport between audience and performers.

> If they don't have that kind of confidence in you, and you don't have the confidence in yourself, then something's going to fall. Something's not going to quite connect.

The authenticity of the characters, combined with excellent performance skills and perhaps the proximity of performances being delivered in non-theatre spaces, sometimes led audience members to sustain their belief in characters after the play had finished and the yarning circle commenced. Isaac Drandic suggested that in *Chopped Liver*, many audience members assumed that he and the other actors shared the same truths and life stories as the characters they were playing. He highlighted how this created a safe space, enabling audiences to open up and speak more candidly about their personal experiences with hepatitis C and other issues. Melodie Reynolds-Diarra agreed: "A lot of the time they thought that that was us on stage; that was our story. … So we got a lot of people's medical history and personal stuff of how they'd gotten [hep C] as well." Shannon Hood described a similar experience in *Viral*.

> One of the Elders actually thought I had hep C and I was like, no, no, I was just acting. I don't have it, it's okay, I'm healthy. [Laughs] Yeah, she looked pretty relieved to find out that I didn't have it.

Conclusion

In addition to these most frequently cited aspects of performance aesthetics in the health education works, practitioners and audience members recognised additional elements such as set design, music, and energy/pace/tempo as being important. Like many touring educational productions, the majority of the works had minimal set design and props, relying instead on the skills of performers and the power of the writing to carry the stories. In *Chopped Liver*, the set consisted of five red boxes that were arranged in various formations to represent different objects and worlds. As described in Chap. 2, the *Viral* set was more symbolic and featured an original score, composed by small sound, that included theme songs for each character, elevating the production values to a level beyond its predecessors and providing another strong point of engagement for audiences. The elements described in this chapter therefore all contributed to the strength of these works as gripping yarns that first and foremost engaged and entertained audiences in the emotional arc and journeys of characters who were specifically drawn to reflect the complexity and diversity of Aboriginal and Torres Strait Islander communities. The sophistication of the works was integral to their power in deftly walking the line between entertainment and education, effectively promoting audience engagement and connection, and supporting the health education and messaging while also speaking to the wider social and political contexts within which such health inequities exist. As such, we argue that they sit comfortably within the wider canon of contemporary First Nations theatre in Australia, making a compelling contribution to dramaturgies of strength, wellbeing, and resistance. These ideas are further developed in the next chapter, where we discuss the third and final theme within our study, examining how the works engaged audiences in the health messaging and information and created culturally safe spaces for challenging stigma and promoting community empowerment and self-determination.

References

Bell-Wykes, Kamarra. 2018a. *Chopped Liver*. Hobart: Australian Script Centre Inc. (trading as AustralianPlays.org).

———. 2018b. *North West of Nowhere*. Hobart: Australian Script Centre Inc. (trading as AustralianPlays.org).

Boal, Augusto. 1985. Theatre of the Oppressed. Translated by A. Charles, and Maria-Odilia Leal McBride. New York: Theatre Communications Group.

Brodzinski, Emma. 2010. *Theatre in Health and Care*. Springer International Publishing.

Cahill, Helen. 2017. Performing the solution: Cautions and Possibilities When Using Theatre Conventions within HIV Prevention Programs. In *Applied Theatre: Performing Health and Wellbeing*, ed. Veronica Baxter and Katharine Low, 145–166. London: Bloomsbury Methuen Drama. https://doi.org/10.5040/9781472584601.ch-006.

Campbell, Alyson, and Jonathan Graffam. 2018. Blood, Shame, Resilience and Hope: Indigenous Theatre Maker Jacob Boehme's *Blood on the Dance Floor*. In *Viral Dramaturgies: HIV and AIDS in Performance in the Twenty-First Century*, ed. Alyson Campbell and Dirk Gindt, 343–365. Springer International Publishing.

Casey, Maryrose. 2012. Colonisation, Notions of Authenticity and Aboriginal Australian Performance. *Critical Race and Whiteness Studies* 8 (1): 1–18.

———. 2013. Bold, Black, and Brilliant: Aboriginal Australian Drama. In *A Companion to Australian Aboriginal Literature*, ed. Belinda Wheeler, 155–172. Boydell & Brewer. http://www.jstor.org/stable/10.7722/j.ctt31njb6.15=Copy.

Cooper, Chris. 2013. The performer in TIE. In *Learning Through Theatre*, ed. A. Anthony Jackson and Chris Vine, 145–155. Routledge.

Hurley, Angelina. 2015. What's So Funny About Aboriginal and Torres Strait Islander Humour? *The Conversation*, March 12. https://theconversation.com/profiles/angelina-hurley-144095/articles

Ilbijerri Theatre Company. 2013. *Annual Report*. Melbourne: Ilbijerri Theatre Company. Supplied.

———. 2014. *Annual Report*. Melbourne: Ilbijerri Theatre Company. Supplied.

Keating, Clare. 2009. *'Chopped Liver' Evaluation Report*. Effective Change Pty Ltd. Melbourne: Ilbijerri Theatre Company. Supplied.

Miller, Elaine, Heidi J. Bergmeier, Claire Blewitt, Amanda O'Connor, and Helen Skouteris. 2021. A Systematic Review of Humour-based Strategies for Addressing Public Health Priorities. *Australian and New Zealand Journal of Public Health* 45 (6): 568–577.

Scar Trees. 2019. By Declan Furber Gillick. Adapted by Kamarra Bell-Wykes. Directed by Kamarra Bell-Wykes. Premiered at Northcote Town Hall, Melbourne, Victoria, October 28.

Thorner, Sabra, Fran Edmonds, Maree Clarke, and Paola Balla. 2018. Maree's Backyard: Intercultural Collaborations for Indigenous Sovereignty in Melbourne. *Oceania* 88 (3): 269–291. https://doi.org/10.1002/ocea.5206.

Viral – Are You the Cure? 2018. By Maryann Sam. Directed by Kamarra Bell-Wykes. Various sites throughout Victoria, 2018–2019.

Welsh, Blayne. 2018. The Hepatitis C Trilogy: A Case for Indigenous Theatre as a Contemporary Manifestation of Traditional Healing Business. *Australasian Drama Studies* 73: 20–41. https://search.informit.org/doi/abs/10.3316/ielapa.146479491877297.

Wilson, Shawn. 2008. *Research is Ceremony: Indigenous Research Methods.* Fernwood.

CHAPTER 6

Stigma-Free Spaces for Healing, Empowerment, and Self-Determination

Abstract This chapter presents further findings from our study on the five health education works led by Kamarra Bell-Wykes and produced by Ilbijerri Theatre Company from 2006 to 2019. These findings draw on interviews conducted with eight practitioners who were involved over the years as performers, production staff, and advisors, a research yarn conducted between co-authors Sarah and Kamarra, and Kamarra's own critical reflections while putting together this volume. We also analysed documents and data from Ilbijerri's corporate archive and published works such as those by Clare Keating (*'Chopped Liver' Evaluation Report*. Effective Change Pty Ltd. Melbourne: Ilbijerri Theatre Company. Supplied, 2009) and Blayne Welsh (The Hepatitis C Trilogy: A Case for Indigenous Theatre as a Contemporary Manifestation of Traditional Healing Business. *Australasian Drama Studies* 73: 20–41. https://search.informit.org/doi/abs/10.3316/ielapa.146479491877297, 2018). This chapter explores the third of three prominent themes within the data: how the works engaged audiences in the health messaging and information and created culturally safe spaces for challenging stigma and promoting community empowerment and self-determination. As such, we continue to argue that the works progress the dramaturgies of wellbeing, strength, and resistance that characterise contemporary First Nations theatre in Australia.

S. Woodland, K. Bell-Wykes, *First Nations Australian Theatre for Health Equity*, https://doi.org/10.1007/978-3-031-65506-7_6

Keywords First Nations theatre • Theatre in education • Applied theatre • Arts and health • Theatre for health education

The previous chapter discusses the aesthetic and performative elements of the health education works in terms of their function as 'gripping dramatic yarns.' We now discuss how this enabled the works to artfully walk a line between entertainment and education, effectively promoting audience engagement and connection and supporting the health education and messaging. Perhaps more importantly, the culturally centred storytelling also created safe spaces that challenged stigma and supported movement towards collective empowerment and healing. We discuss how the performances invited audiences to take control of their own lives and wellbeing and to be inspired and filled with a sense of pride at seeing their own stories and lives represented on stage. The findings also point towards the importance of these works in building the skills and capacities of audience members, community members, health workers, performers, and creatives, both in learning about and addressing the health issues but also in terms of transforming their own lives, 'giving back', and adopting community leadership roles. This reflects the need for the work to address change at the structural level, as opposed to only focusing on individual behaviours (Low 2017). As such, we continue to argue that the works progress the dramaturgies of wellbeing, strength, and resistance that characterise contemporary First Nations theatre in Australia, as discussed in Chap. 3.

Audience Engagement and Connection

The previous chapter demonstrates how audiences were strongly engaged by the performance aesthetics in the health education plays, which speaks to their power, not only as standalone theatre works but also in terms of their capacity to deliver health messaging and education goals. A critical element in the success of the performances in engaging audiences—as is the case with most applied theatre—was that they were toured into communities as opposed to mainstream theatres, largely meeting audience members *where they were*. Isaac Drandic attributed *Chopped Liver*'s success to this: "Going to the communities is a big one, going to them rather than anybody coming to us. In the city, it's hard to get people through the doors" (interview, 2021). Jesse Butler described how impactful it was to tour *Viral* into communities in terms of them being the "right audiences" for the work:

> You're going to make ten times the impact if people understand the story and they can relate to it, and they understand what's going on and they're going through it maybe themselves. … This is why we get sick of performing in front of those audiences that we know it's not for because you're just like, I feel like I'm wasting an hour here. I should be performing in front of people who are going to get something from this. (Interview, 2020)

As health worker and reference group member Peter Waples-Crowe observed, this presents some challenges in terms of the cost of mounting tours, which can result in performances having limited reach and therefore limited impact (interview, 2021). Nevertheless, over the past fifteen years, Ilbijerri's health education performances have reached over 26,000 audience members in a wide variety of community settings, and findings from the data suggest that these performances have been highly engaging.

While it is impossible to gauge the long-term effects of the performances on individual and community health, as will be discussed further below, evidence suggests that the immediacy and liveness of a theatre performance create a unique affective response that supports the continued use of theatre in this context. As discussed widely in the literature, live theatre possesses specific qualities that highlight its potential as a unique vehicle for health education and messaging. In the context of a community event, theatre's liveness, energy, and emotional intensity (when done well) lends itself to critical, dialogic, collective meaning making and experiential learning in ways that often transcend what is possible through other artforms such as visual art or recorded video (Brodzinski 2010; Cahill 2017; Campbell and Gindt 2018; Low 2017; Prendergast and Saxton 2016). These qualities certainly are not found in more traditional approaches to health education and messaging, such as pamphlets and seminars. As Melodie Reynolds-Diarra observed:

> That's the magic of live storytelling … you're sharing the same air space as these people that you're telling the story to. … I think it vibrates and stays with people longer and in more layers of them when there is someone live in front of you [and] the one-to-one contact of looking in someone's eyes and going through something onstage, [as] opposed to looking into a television's eyes, or a movie's eyes. … There's that humanisation of, 'Hey, it's okay, we're all going through it too, but here's us helping each other.' (Interview, 2021)

Melodie describes here the relationality that is at the heart of these works' power as 'gripping yarns', where audiences could identify and connect with the characters and stories on stage in a visceral sense, becoming part of a community of people on a journey together towards healing.

Nevertheless, our research shows that some audiences were more engaged than others, echoing Jesse's earlier assertion that the works needed to find the "right audience." As discussed in Chap. 5, when *Viral* was toured to schools, there were sometimes lower levels of engagement from audiences. Performer Shannon Hood put this down to a potential lack of experience with the themes and issues being presented, and Jesse Butler suggested that a factor in this may have been the sheer size of the audiences and the fact that school students were less likely to let down their guard. However, there is overwhelming evidence that prison audiences were among the most highly engaged, particularly for tours of *Chopped Liver* and *Viral*. Blayne Welsh (2018, 31) observed,

> Throughout the comedic moments, but also in the emotionally intense and sad moments, there was constant laughter from inmates at each of the correctional centres. The inmates made for a very engaged audience. During the yarning circles held afterwards, they were also highly expressive and very respectful.

Both Isaac Drandic and Melodie Reynolds-Diarra described how prison audience members' body language would change as they let their guard down throughout the performance of *Chopped Liver*. Melodie recalled:

> They'd start like this with their arms folded. It's like they completely blocked off, they didn't want to be there. … Within the first couple of minutes their arms, their body language completely changed, and they were engaged in the work.

Melodie vividly described how this also extended to the prison guards, highlighting the power of the performance to break down the hostile division between "prisoners" and "screws":

> There was, I think, 160 inmates and that's the first time that they'd had all those all inmates in one area ever, so there was about 60 guards … all standing in a semicircle around the back. … All of them were just scanning the group, not even paying attention to us setting up or starting or anything like

> that. I remember the … feeling the tension in the room. It was just like, 'Whoa!' … So you had this tension on both sides and then you had us—like, me, Isaac, and PJ [tour manager] all tense like that too because of all this but, no, just go ahead with the story. I remember about ten minutes, 15 minutes into it and then I looked up … I saw the screws' faces; well, their arms had dropped, like so they weren't crossed, and they were looking at us. … They were focussed on the story that was happening … and they weren't looking at the inmates because they noticed as well that the inmates weren't focussed on each other … they were just focussed on the story. I was like, 'Wow!' … that's some pretty honest and raw writing and [the] way that the performance was put together as well that made that happen, that could even capture that attention from such hard-core military almost, kind of energy into, 'No, I'm going to listen to this yarn here.'

By taking performances into prisons and other community sites, these works also engaged many first-time theatregoers. Nazaree Dickerson described how this was one of the things she enjoyed: "I always love it when you hear somebody from the audience say that's the first theatre show I've ever seen. That is just something that blows me away" (interview, 2021). Peter Waples-Crowe echoed this sentiment: "The people I brought along to *Chopped Liver* more recently, it just made their day to see Aboriginal people up there, acting. They probably never get exposed to theatre that way, it's really important." To counteract some of the traditionally held expectations of silence and composure in viewing theatre, performances included a preamble or set of protocols for the audience to follow so that they felt they had permission to call out or respond. This cut through some of the awkwardness of performing in small spaces and invited audience members to engage more freely. As outlined in the tour notes from *Viral*:

> We found that it changed the atmosphere for the better when we got Mary [stage/tour manager] to announce that it was okay to laugh, cry and respond to the work, as for a lot of the audiences, it was their first time seeing a performance. The start was always a little tense as they weren't sure how to act within the performance context. We found that once we'd announce this, the audience would get straight into the performance as it released the mental stress of how to receive the work. Mary forgot to do this at one of the performances and they were really tense for the first ten minutes because they didn't know to react to the stimuli. (Tour Notes – Improvements for next time! n.d.)

Another key audience for the works was professionals working in the health and social sectors, where performances were delivered at conferences. These performances have invariably received high praise (often standing ovations), with delegates finding them a highly innovative and entertaining way to impart health information and education. Shannon Hood reflected on how fulfilling it had been for him to perform in this context: "A lot of people came up and thanked us for the performance and that sort of thing. Yeah, I thought that was the highlight" (interview, 2021). This finding has implications for building professional capacity within the health and social care sectors, as will be discussed later, drawing workers into the emotional truths and complexities of the health concerns being explored.

Everyone who contributed to this study acknowledged that not all the health education performances were equally engaging for audiences, sometimes with different factors at play in influencing the levels of engagement. Kamarra reflected that the differences between *Chopped Liver*, *North West of Nowhere*, and *Body Armour* had to do with the energy of the plays.

> It was something to do with the pace of the story telling, and I think that first of all, *Body Armor* had all these scenes in the doctor's office, which were awful. It was death on stage, and it became a 'performed pamphlet,' which we'll never do again. However, then *North West of Nowhere*, even though people enjoyed it, it was a much softer yarn and it was a much slower kind of yarn. I think that … wasn't received as well as *Chopped Liver* … and *Viral*, because of that. Therefore, … you've got to have some fast—you've got to grab people. You've got to get in there at a truly high energy to captivate harder to engage audiences like teenagers and prisoners, although this would be different when creating work for say Elders. (Interview, 2021)

Kamarra discussed with Jesse Butler how *North West of Nowhere* was perhaps less engaging than *Viral*, particularly in terms of the target audience of young people. Echoing comments cited earlier, Jesse suggested that the audience may have felt awkward with the material, "But you kind of hope that you kind of are just planting seeds, and just reiterating to people what is important and also with blackfullas, you know, like we're not forgetting you." Kamarra suggested that this may have also been due to the development of the piece, which, with an outside director, unlike *Viral*, had not been built from the ground up through community workshops. As discussed elsewhere, over the course of the five productions,

Kamarra became aware that with higher levels of community engagement from the outset, there would be higher levels of audience engagement at the end, informing how she now approaches the health education work, as discussed in our conclusion.

'Walking the Line' Between Entertainment and Education

Integrating the gripping dramatic yarn with appropriate health messaging takes a specific set of creative skills at the writing and development stage so as not to make performances didactic or clunky. The health content in these works was delivered via compelling characters and scenarios, where relationships between people, cultural norms, and wider political contexts were explored, rather than just the pointy end of messages and behaviour. Cahill (2017, 94) suggests that this needs to be approached carefully, as "good theatre can potentially be bad health promotion." She warns against using worst-case scenarios as central subject matter, as this is akin to fear tactics. Furthermore, using stock characters and good/bad binaries can exacerbate stigma and connect illness to moral character. Kamarra's approach has always instinctively followed this advice, with the conviction that the plays are never only about the health issues but also about the emotional, social, and political contexts surrounding them. By asking, "What is the play *really* about?" (see Chap. 2), Kamarra pushed the performances beyond being "performed pamphlets" and into meaningful narratives of transformation. Not only does this deepen the nuance of the interrogation from an educational perspective, but it also enables stronger aesthetic engagement from a wider audience that may include friends, family, health workers, and others. As discussed elsewhere, this impacted Kamarra herself and other creatives involved in the works in terms of deepening knowledge of health and wellbeing for themselves and their communities. In this way, Blayne Welsh (2018, 34) argues that educational theatre works such as *Viral* represent "a contemporary form of healing ritual" by extending traditional cultural frameworks and practices to provide a space for all involved—creative teams, performers, and audiences—to engage in a relational exchange of transformative storytelling.

The plays have managed to 'walk the line' between art and education through several deliberate strategies and approaches, sometimes in tension with requests from funding bodies, who sometimes want facts and information to be delivered in dry, obvious ways. Kamarra recalls how the first draft of *Chopped Liver* read like a spoken pamphlet and, as such, died on the creative development floor. She realised that her task was not to inform audiences about the virus but to make them feel something, to make them care enough to seek out their own information and support. She therefore abandoned the alarming but boring statistics and returned to the basic principles of good theatre, truth, emotion, and a good story. *Chopped Liver* needed to deliver a compelling and endearing human story that would open the hearts of the audience, break through stereotypes, and allow practical information to be received. During *Viral*'s development, the community workshops unearthed numerous misconceptions about hep C and its treatment that felt essential to include. To incorporate these different perspectives without overloading the main characters, the team used vox pops, as part of the documentary narrative, as a scene transition device. The actors transformed the "Viragon" set as a chorus of fictional community members, creating a tapestry of voices expressing issue misinformation and stigma.

Actor 1: Think I was immunised against it in school
Actor 2: Hep C? That's like AIDS isn't it?
Actor 3: Can't you catch it from kissing?
Actor 1: Sex?
Actor 2: Mozzies?
Actor 3: Holding hands?
Actor 1: That's why I don't drink out of chipped cups.
Actor 2: It's a junkie's disease isn't it? Dirty junkies.
Actor 3: Waste of space.
Actor 1: Why should our tax dollars pay for their treatment?
All: Scum! (*Viral - Are You the Cure?* 2018)

For Kamarra, one of the reasons *Body Armour* was less successful, both artistically and educationally, was the inclusion of a doctor's office where most of the play was set and where the piece didactically delivered facts and statistics.

Doc: And your 'old man' is hepatitis C positive?
Harley: He's dead positive.
Doc: Oh, I'm assuming he had chronic hepatitis C for some time then?
Harley: He was sick. How do I know if it was the virus, the drugs, or the grog?
Doc: Most likely a combination of all three.

Harley: Towards the end his skin had this yellow tinge; like smoker's fingers, a walking nicotine stain. And his eyes, you know when you take a leak, and your piss hits the water, spreads like smoke—muddy yellow mist. That's what his eyes looked like, like toilet water tainted with piss. (Bell-Wykes 2018a)

Despite all attempts to maintain the artistic integrity of the work, this device came as a direct request from a reference group member at considerable cost to the artistic integrity of the work. The play crossed the line into pamphlet territory to the detriment of the art, the audience, and ultimately the health message. Peter Waples-Crowe observed that in his role in the Aboriginal Community Controlled Health Organisation (ACCHO) space, "You are often at loggerheads with the Department of Health anyway. They have a set of performance indicators they want to meet, and they're very bureaucratic." For Peter, handing the reins to Kamarra as the lead creative made perfect sense: "She's the expert in this field."

Walking the line for Kamarra has meant sometimes digging more deeply into the issue than simply delivering information about how to be safe or healthy. In *North West of Nowhere*, the Department of Health wanted to promote the new contraceptive implant Implanon as a way of promoting safe sex. Kamarra was conscious, however, that this did not negate the possibility of contracting STIs, and she had been made aware that in some communities, boys were rubbing girls' arms to see if they had a rod in a kind of courting gesture. She therefore included this in the script, providing the audience with more nuance on the topic than an uncritical promotional message would. The works have also maintained their artistic integrity through finding creative solutions to explore the various health topics in interesting but appropriate ways. A sexual interaction between Nella and Cuz in *North West of Nowhere* was demonstrated via a text-driven, stylised dance demonstrating consent and the negotiation of safe sex, offering the characters' internal perspectives and poetically elevating the performance (Fig. 6.1).

Nella: A smile, a smell, a wink, a wave, eyes meet, hold for a moment, shyly look away.

Cuz: A whisper, a wiggle in her hips, guards are down, sexy lick of the lips.

Nella: Flirting, dancing, hands touch for a beat, instant connection, a certain type of heat. (Bell-Wykes 2018b)

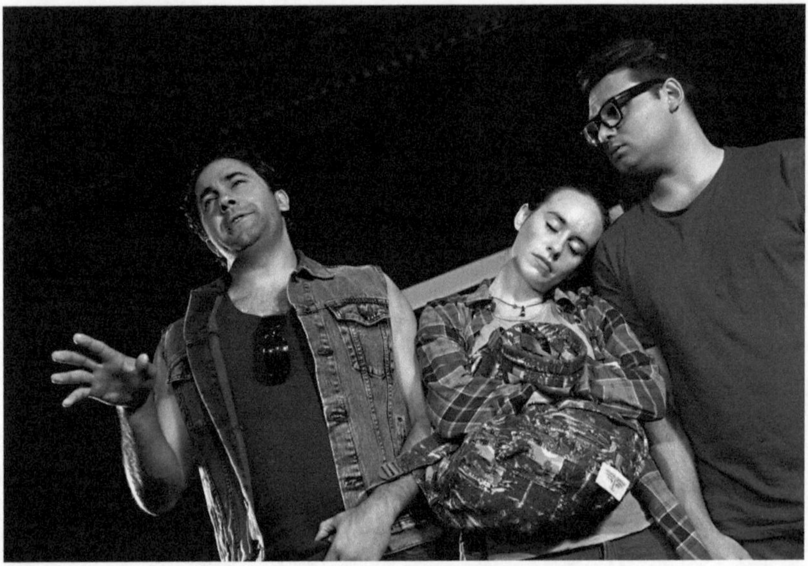

Fig. 6.1 (L-R) James Henry, Shaynee Brayshaw, and Ian Michael, *North West of Nowhere*. Image by Stephen Rhall (2014)

Such artistic decisions also extended to exploring the wider systemic, political, and community contexts in which health issues exist. For example, 'White Spirit' branded kerosene cans were incorporated into the scene transformations of *Viral*, symbolising the infiltration of the colonial virus infecting the worlds of the characters (and the audience). This theme was again expressed by the community workshop participants, and Kamarra was determined to acknowledge and represent it through the piece. Audience feedback in the guest book for *Viral* (2018) directly reflected how successfully these works were able to walk the line between aesthetics and health messaging:

> Great performance – dance sequence profound. Will distribute health materials to our Mob.
>
> Such an amazingly powerful show, I learnt heaps!!
>
> So powerfully done. So illustrated the barriers and complexities to taking up treatment.
>
> Thank you so much, very deep, heart-warming, and informative.

Very touching performance but with lots of education.

Absolutely amazing performance. Very touching and informative. Thank you.

Great show, it was a great way to put the message across in an accessible way.

Stigma-Free Space for Yarning

The quality of the works as dramatic yarns was integral to their function in breaking stigma and opening a safe space for open talk or yarning about personal experiences and connections to the content. Even in cases prior to *Viral*, where performers may have felt rushed on tours, delivering multiple shows per day in a variety of settings, in most cases, there remained high levels of audience engagement and community connection, leading audience members to share their own personal experiences, sometimes for the first time in yarning circles afterwards. Isaac Drandic suggested that the quality of *Chopped Liver* as a piece of theatre enabled the actors to earn the trust of the audience so that they would be more receptive to the pamphlets that were ultimately handed out at the end (Fig. 6.2). This sentiment was echoed by Kamarra and Laila Thaker in their conversation about *Viral*:

Laila: You could see them loosening up through the show so probably by the time we did get to the yarning circle … from what I observed it seemed like … they'd been given themselves permission to just…

Kamarra: To let their guard down.

Laila: Yeah. (Interview, 2021)

Dramaturgies of strength, wellbeing, and resistance in contemporary First Nations theatre often work to challenge the shames and stigmas imposed by colonisation. The 'colonial load' of negative connotations around poor health as signifying poverty, neglect, or 'dirtiness' has been projected through the mainstream media and culture in Australia since colonisation. Intergenerational trauma impacts such as family violence and drug and alcohol dependence are also shrouded in a sense of shame for many Aboriginal and Torres Strait Islander communities, where the blame for such wellbeing issues is wrongly laid at their feet. Nazaree Dickerson highlighted the important role of theatre in counteracting this sense of blame, shame, and stigma:

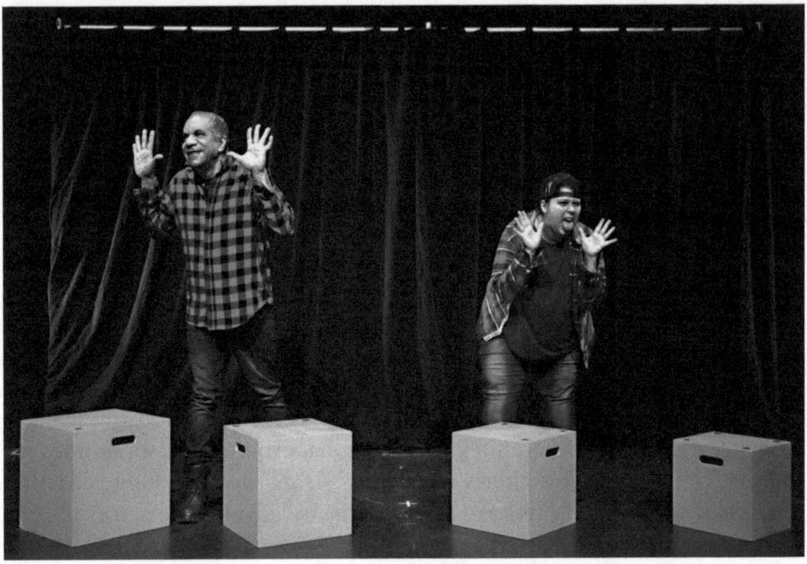

Fig. 6.2 Gregory J. Fryer (L) and Nazaree Dickerson (R), *Chopped Liver*. Image by James Henry (2017)

> Theatre's such a wonderful way of bringing people together to discuss things that sometimes don't get discussed in … community forums, without it being about a blame game. It is actually about … just safely discussing something.

In her report on *Chopped Liver*, Keating (2009, 17) cited an audience member in observing how the play broke down stigma "through accessible, real, funny characters and a story that you believe" and "humanising hepatitis C so that it is no longer this scary, dirty thing, but a fact of life." She went on to highlight that "from the perspective of [partner organisation] Hepatitis C Victoria, having anywhere from 20 to 300 people laughing and chatting about hepatitis C is a major achievement" (19). For Kamarra, the significance was much greater, breaking down years of historical stigma and providing a sense of relief among audience members at finally being given "permission" to talk about hep C.

> At the time that *Chopped Liver* was commissioned, it was one of the dirtiest words and there was so much shame. There was, nobody was talking about

> it. People didn't know what it was, the rates of it were so high. So suddenly when you got that, started getting named on stage and jokes were being made and emotional truths were being identified about that experience. The permission that was kind of given to these audience members that had been holding this shame inside them for so long, it was almost like a floodgate was being opened.

Health worker Peter Waples-Crowe described how these levels of shame and stigma contributed to misinformation and "urban myths," which could only be challenged through honest, unflinching examination of the issue and surrounding behaviours. In relation to the depiction of injecting drugs, he was adamant:

> Let's not shy away from it. It is one of the biggest methods for transmitting blood borne viruses, like hep C and HIV. For our communities, sometimes we don't want to bring more shame on our community, and I can see why people feel that. But I feel we have to name and make it realistic, and I think that's what the plays do, they don't steer away from it.

Shannon Hood observed how important the freedom to discuss the virus safely enabled audience members at *Viral* to learn about the new safe and simple oral treatment for hep C and take this information back to their communities: "They were like, 'Oh yeah, well my niece has got it,' or, 'My daughter has got it,' or, 'My son's got it and we didn't even know that there was a treatment for it'" (interview, 2021).

This is reflected in the literature, where we see that there is often a palpable sense of relief in audiences when a stigmatising topic is presented with compassion rather than judgement. In discussing the performance *Sexwise* in Aotearoa, New Zealand, Trish Wells (2013) tracks significant positive responses from both students and teachers around the affective impact on students, including the pleasure (and relief) of dialogue around these topics. Jacob Boehme also reflected on how his performance *Blood on the Dancefloor* prompted audience members to approach him privately to discuss the impact of HIV in their families and communities (Campbell and Graffam 2018, 363). Campbell and Gindt (2018, 28) describe how the communality created by an ephemeral performance can then lead to a "viral" spreading of conversation and engagement beyond the life of the performance, inviting the wider community to engage with the complexity of lived experience and the associated stigma.

When *Chopped Liver* was first toured, there was no formal yarning or debrief with the audience built into performances with this happening organically over food and drink as described by Isaac above. During this conversation with Isaac, Kamarra recalled being shocked by how this occurred in the prison setting, describing it as a "confessional" where people were sharing deeply personal experiences of the virus. After this first tour of *Chopped Liver*, the need became evident for a more formal, facilitated yarning circle after performances, where people would be invited to reflect on the performances. Jesse Butler articulated the importance of this process from a cultural perspective:

> The yarning circles weren't there to talk about how great we are or how good this message is. It was about breaking down … all the stigma and breaking down everything that we put up and just getting rid of it, and sitting in a circle which is what blackfullas do. We sit in a circle, and we yarn and we're honest. Then, we perform in front of each other, and we talk about stuff. … Therefore, it's not just sitting in a circle on chairs talking about the kind of health stuff.

In describing how people in the circle "perform in front of each other," Jesse alludes to the times when the yarning circle extended beyond the health issues at hand and created a space where audience members felt they wanted to share their own creative offerings:

> There were a couple of fellas that got up and were like, 'I've prepared this song,' or, 'I've made this thing.' So, all of a sudden, we opened up this little creative space. People just felt so open. Some people said they can't speak anywhere else, and they spoke to us. … I think that's not just about what they said, but the fact that they could speak in that space to us.

This points towards the holistic function of these works as promoting a sense of positive identity, empowerment, and wellbeing that we discuss further below.

It requires a specific set of skills and capacities to create a safe space for yarning about normally stigmatising issues such as these. Nazaree Dickerson pointed out that this included speaking in "plain language" without using theatre or health jargon and allowing the yarning to be genuine:

> It could easily become a contrived situation where you're trying to control this thing that's meant to be organic, but it is just about actually creating the opportunity for that organic conversation to happen and using plain terms, so that everyone understands.

Kamarra believed that having lived experience of hep C deepened her capacity to lead the yarning circles around that issue, although she acknowledged the high levels of skill that cast members who did not have those experiences also brought to the yarning circles. Another key factor in supporting this process was to ensure, where possible, that a health worker was present to provide accurate information and relieve the performers of this burden. A further layer of safety was provided in the yarning circles by performers and creative teams managing input from non-Indigenous audience members. Mary Quinsacara recalled how in one performance of the *Viral* tour, the decision was made to dispense with the yarning circle, as there were some non-Indigenous folks in the audience who were at risk of dominating the conversation (interview, 2020). Nazaree Dickerson explained that for First Nations audiences, the presence of non-Indigenous members in the yarning circle can lead to self-censorship.

> If you're someone that - from the community that doesn't necessarily speak or articulate yourself in a polite way, you're just going to shut your mouth rather than swear in front of these nice white people that you don't really know to tell your story.

While these works did not exclude non-Indigenous audiences, First Nations voices were given priority so that the space itself did not become colonised. Kamarra was clear, however, that in sector-related shows, non-Indigenous health workers and other professionals could be invited to unpack issues through yarning, as this formed an important part of their professional development, as discussed further below.

Delivering the Health Messages

Notwithstanding a commitment to artfulness and theatricality in these performances, Kamarra always maintained a strong focus on the brief of delivering the key overall health messages and information that were being sought by health partners and advisors, albeit in conversation with the wider systemic and political drivers of ill health among Aboriginal and Torres Strait Islander communities. As discussed elsewhere, the messaging was contextualised and deepened in *Viral* through community consultation, dialogue, and collaboration with the people directly affected by the issues, reflecting best practice in Aboriginal and Torres Strait Islander health (Gee et al. 2014) as well as theatre for health education (Brodzinski 2010; Low 2017, 2020). Furthermore, as discussed in Chap. 5, their aesthetic framing as culturally informed yarns provided an anti-oppressive framework for imparting the health information. Our literature review highlighted the shortcomings in evaluating the success of theatre-based programs such as these, and several authors discuss how difficult it is (perhaps impossible) to credit such interventions directly with positive health outcomes, especially in the longer term (Brodzinski 2010; Prendergast and Saxton 2016). Emma Brodzinski (2010) notes the trend in arts and health to place high value on evidencing results and the tensions of working between traditions of empirical data in the sciences and qualitative data in the arts (a perceived polarity that is often stereotypical and inaccurate on both sides, as she clarifies). Traditional "post program" evaluation tools such as those used by Ilbijerri and other arts organisations, while helpful in making the case for continued funding, can sometimes have shortcomings in capturing meaningful data that might give a fuller picture of the work's efficacy. We are currently attempting to address this tension through our latest project, *The Score*, as discussed in the conclusion.

Despite these tensions, Ilbijerri's archive of evaluation data and reporting at least provides a snapshot of the positive impact of the works on audience members. Audience survey data for *Viral* (2018 and 2019) and *Scar Trees* (2019) indicate that the plays raised understanding of the issues, promoted help-seeking behaviours, challenged stigma, and therefore may have contributed to overcoming barriers to treatment or support (see Tables 6.1 and 6.2).

The *Chopped Liver* report highlights how, in some cases, audiences already knew the information being imparted, but the play functioned as a compelling reminder to seek testing and treatment.

> In the male prisons, we've moved beyond the prevention message because it seems like just about everyone has it, but the play is a wake up and reminder call. I have had prisoners ask detailed questions because they haven't known about testing. (Kirk Peterson, Victorian Prisons Program Educator, as reported in Keating 2009, 7)

Table 6.1 Data gathered from Viral performances (2018, 2019) using the Culture Counts survey platform

Viral	*2018 93 audience members surveyed*	*2019 51 audience members surveyed*
Viral gave me an insight into the difficulty some people have accessing health care.	66% strongly agreed[a]	87% strongly agreed
Viral helped me understand the stigma and discrimination associated with hepatitis C.	70% strongly agreed	89% strongly agreed
Viral increased my understanding of the prevention, transmission, and treatment of hepatitis C.	67% strongly agreed	75% strongly agreed
I am likely to visit a doctor for a blood test or treatment after watching *Viral* (or suggest to family/friends).	71% said YES	84% said YES

[a]Participants were asked to respond to questions on a Likert scale: strongly agree, agree, neutral, disagree, strongly disagree. For the questions shown in Table 1, no respondents indicated that they strongly disagreed

Table 6.2 Data gathered from Scar Trees performances (2019) using the Culture Counts survey platform

Scar Trees	*2019 48 audience members surveyed*
I now have a greater understanding of where I can go for support if I am, or someone I know is, experiencing family violence.	55% strongly agreed
I feel more confident to take a stand against family violence in my community.	71% strongly agreed
Scar Trees increased my understanding of the barriers faced by First Nations people in reporting family violence.	65% strongly agreed
Scar Trees increased my understanding of different types of family violence.	60% strongly agreed
I feel an increased sense of connection or belonging to my community.	57% strongly agreed

> It provides information – we have to see that as a starting point. But more importantly, it provides a moment of clarity. We sometimes see people literally recognise themselves there. The play reminds them of the need for testing. It reminds those who may even have a diagnosis that it can take a long time before someone becomes symptomatic. I hope it means that people will take the right steps. (Jen Johnson, Australian Research Centre in Sex, Health and Society, as reported in Keating 2009, 8)

Keating (17) also observed that the play promoted positive outcomes from the development of treatments that people may not be aware of. Reports from performances of *Chopped Liver*, *North West of Nowhere*, and *Viral* further highlight how those works prompted audience members to seek help.

> I have had a number of students make appointments to see me about their sexual health after the performance and I am certain it was the production that prompted them to see me and seek advice about STI check-ups and STI prevention. (Secondary School Nurse, Castlemaine, *North West of Nowhere*, Ilbijerri 2015)

Keating (2009, 18) cites Sandra Gregson, a sexual health and blood-borne viruses nurse at the Victorian Aboriginal Health Service (VAHS) who reported having "lots of conversations with people because of *Chopped Liver*. People think about things for a long time. They are happy to ask me questions." Reporting from Viral also demonstrated some positive outcomes for audience members in terms of providing a catalyst for seeking support and testing.

> One person disclosed they had hep C … but didn't follow-through with treatment and we have been able to provide support. (Staff member from Braybrook Community Hub, *Viral* Community Tour Report 2018)

> We had more tested and also we have men talk about hep C more. (Staff member Ravenhall Metropolitan Remand Centre, ibid.)

> Definitely suggesting doctor for others. (Audience comment, Viral 2019 audience survey)

Peter Waples-Crowe discussed the benefit of the plays in promoting conversation, nevertheless acknowledging how difficult it can be to capture these impacts.

> [When] people pull you aside and have a conversation, and I think sometimes the play has probably done that for a lot of people as well and made people think. But we just can't measure that impact, you know. That's one of the impacts we don't know how to measure.

It is often accidental or anecdotal feedback that tells us how effective a program or performance has been. Kamarra vividly recalled a *Chopped*

Liver audience member recognising her at the local shops after seeing one of the shows while serving time and joyfully calling out, "Hey you're the one that came inside with the hep C show!" A handful of prisoners on long-term sentences testified to seeing all the plays, affectionally expressing a clear investment in the work, discussing their favourite characters, and asking about actors from past tours.

Community Empowerment and Self-Determination

The impacts reported in the evaluations, although somewhat limited in terms of rigorous and artful research design, indicate the possibility that audience members were prompted towards developing positive behaviours and attitudes that might support their own and others' wellbeing. Nevertheless, as suggested by the range of literature we have explored for this study, health and wellbeing outcomes in projects such as these can be seen as "much richer and more complex than mere behaviour change" (Low 2020, 15). While the findings cited above around health education and challenging stigma for audiences are extremely promising, through the process of developing and touring these works and the spaces for yarning that were created, there was potential for much deeper engagement that could promote empowerment, capacity building, and wellbeing in a broader sense.

An important but underreported outcome from projects such as these is the potential for them to develop the skills and capacities of performers and creative teams (beyond performance skills, as discussed in Chap. 5), empowering them to strengthen their own health and wellbeing and to become advocates and facilitators for change in their communities. Several creative team members we interviewed described how being involved in these works was rewarding, reinforcing their resolve to give back to their communities and strengthening their skills in working responsively, ethically, and flexibly with community participants and audiences. As discussed in Chap. 5, Jesse Butler talked about how being involved in *Viral* opened his eyes to how performance could be and do so much more than what he had previously experienced in mainstream theatre. Laila Thaker also reflected on how educational theatre enabled her to give back to her community and make "meaningful change." She cited *Viral* as one of the most "memorable" productions she had been involved in. "I learnt a lot from that project and definitely it's just made me a better person." She went on to describe how this was an important legacy work for her:

> You don't want to give up on the project or the community because it's bigger than you, you've got to put yourself aside and understand that - keep coming back to the bigger picture. Next generation stuff. You're doing it for the next generation so it's easier.

In terms of direct health and wellbeing outcomes for creative teams, Kamarra herself highlighted how the process of writing *Chopped Liver* supported her in her own hep C journey: "I came to really give myself an education about the virus. … I started managing the virus better and undoubtedly improved my own personal health outcomes and emotional trajectory around the virus." At the start of the creative development for *Viral*, because none of the other ensemble members had lived experience of hep C, Kamarra asked the team to write down everything they knew about the virus, including any stereotypes and misconceptions. Laila Thaker described how this enabled her to "unpack and rip open" the stigma, providing a collective starting point before engaging with the facts and emotional truths explored in the play. By participating in the creative development and the community workshops that informed the work, the creative team entered their own process of challenging stigma and educating themselves about the virus.

Perhaps the most compelling example of this was in the case of Shannon Hood, who drew on his own parallel lived experiences of addiction and rehabilitation to inform his roles in *Viral* while also developing his skills in performance and community engagement. Shannon related how he drew on his personal experience of recovery to respond to the unfamiliar demands of performing and touring.

> It's very challenging and it's a big commitment. Probably the biggest commitment I've made in the last couple of years. … What I'd overcome [with addiction] I thought was a lot bigger and a lot harder to do than actually getting through a three-week tour or a six-week tour doing a theatrical play. I kept telling myself, this is a lot easier, there's no withdrawal. You might be missing this, or you don't have time to do that and that. Thought about drinking, thought about smoking, rah, rah. Yeah, just hav[e] to keep your mind concentrated on what you've committed yourself to and basically at the end of the tour what you would have accomplished in a personal sense and then in a community sense, as well.

While this was at times challenging for him and his fellow cast members, Kamarra saw his development as equally important as the show and the audience experience. In her view, Shannon's involvement as an inexperienced actor but identifiable community member contributed to raising aspirations in community audiences, encouraging them to imagine taking the stage and adopting a similar leadership role, prompting her to develop this approach in the current project *The Score* in ways that would deepen the wellbeing impacts by building capacity in communities.

> After seeing Shannon on stage … dropping lines, making mistakes, having a laugh, just keeping on going. … For the first time people said, 'I reckon I could do that. I want to do that.' Our audiences never said that before. They would say, 'Amazing performers, wow, they're so amazing. Wow, how do you do that? I could never do that; how do you do that?' So that was another important revelation to wanting to move this work in that direction.

Shannon described the power of this from his perspective, highlighting his role as a peer mentor within his community:

> For me, to be up on stage and committing and doing a performance, I was hoping it would send the message to certain people - and even the lads in the jail and that sort of thing. They know my history too, a few of them. A couple of my cousins came up and said to me, 'Mate, I'm proud of you. From when I saw you a few years ago, mate, I would never have thought this was possible. I thought you would have been in here, been in the greens [prison uniform], not in a performance mate.' That was a massive incentive to me to continue and try and just let a few lads out there know that change is very possible.

Speaking more broadly, Jesse Butler discussed how First Nations stories are not told enough in the mainstream and that with more representation, more First Nations peoples might become involved in creative programs and projects. Peter Waples-Crowe also described how the works might impact audiences in this way:

> I just know some of the Aboriginal people I work with just found the whole experience really life affirming, and yeah, just seeing themselves reflected and seeing such excellence, and how deadly it all was. … I think sometimes we're pushed to the margins and seeing us at the forefront and doing innovative stuff is really good. I think it just counteracts a lot of negative narratives. … Maybe it inspires people in the audience to go into acting, you know, maybe they see a potential for themselves. … Or you know, they might want to work in that area.

In her report on *Chopped Liver*, Keating (2009, 16) described how empowerment for audiences has always been on Kamarra's agenda as a writer.

> Because the play is so powerful and the acting is so strong and the play concludes on such a positive ending, those who have toured with the play say that at the end, the sense of pride of Indigenous audience members is palpable. …This response is exactly what was intended by playwright Kamarra Bell-Wykes, who observed that 'these (young guys) don't get that sense of pride very often – it just doesn't happen when you are so marginalized. But I've seen the young guys watch this and puff out with pride at the end – that is really special. That's exactly what I wanted to do.'"

Despite having such intentions towards empowerment and affirmation for audiences, the experience of touring *Scar Trees* demonstrated that this was not always a given in these performances. Kamarra observed that while it was well received by the arts community, the tour should have focused on perpetrators or professionals and policy makers rather than victim-survivors:

> It felt like there wasn't really any empowerment for the victims. … It just kind of felt like there was a bit of a retriggering process that was going on and I don't know whether it was for the right people or not.

Nazaree Dickerson agreed that it was possible that audiences were "left with these wounds that have maybe been reopened and we don't know." For a performance focusing on family violence, this was certainly not an ideal outcome. The funding body, reference group, partner organisations, Ilbijerri team, and Kamarra all underestimated the impact of the show and failed to adequately interrogate who it was for and why, leading to this significant oversight. For Kamarra, this highlighted the importance of maintaining strong community consultation and engagement at all stages and establishing clear and appropriate goals for projects, a lesson that she again carried into her more recent work.

The presentation of the works at conferences and other professional development settings such as Aboriginal Community Controlled Health Organisations (ACCHOS) was also an important step in widening the impacts of the work, building capacity for health and social care workers to understand the complexities of the issues beyond behaviour change and for health leaders to discuss strategies for meeting specific challenges (Keating 2009, 18). As Peter Waples-Crowe stated in the Community Tour Report for *Viral* (2018):

> It also left an impression on the Thorne Harbour Health Staff who attended and strengthened our relationships and their knowledge of hep C and Aboriginal theatre. A cultural awareness raising exercise for the mainstream mob in the audience.

Conclusion

This chapter demonstrates that the health education works operated in multiple ways to achieve holistic outcomes in wellbeing beyond simply imparting health information and messaging or promoting behaviour change. The data suggest that witnessing their own stories and experiences portrayed on stage filled audience members with "life-affirming" pride and aspiration. Furthermore, the plays nurtured the skills and capabilities of various stakeholders—audience members, community members, health professionals, performers, and creatives—to not only acquire knowledge about health issues but also undergo personal development and transformations that might ripple out into the wider community. However, as we conclude in the next chapter, Kamarra acknowledges that unlocking this potential requires a deeper and more sustained level of community engagement within the projects. The journey towards meaningful change continues, with the theatre serving as a powerful catalyst for both personal growth and collective transformation.

References

———. 2018a. *Body Armour*. Hobart: Australian Script Centre Inc. (trading as AustralianPlays.org).

———. 2018b. *North West of Nowhere*. Hobart: Australian Script Centre Inc. (trading as AustralianPlays.org).

Brodzinski, Emma. 2010. *Theatre in Health and Care*. Springer International Publishing.

Cahill, Helen. 2017. Performing the Solution: Cautions and Possibilities When Using Theatre Conventions within HIV Prevention Programs. In *Applied Theatre: Performing Health and Wellbeing*, ed. Veronica Baxter and Katharine Low, 145–166. London: Bloomsbury Methuen Drama. https://doi.org/10.5040/9781472584601.ch-006.

Campbell, Alyson, and Dirk Gindt. 2018. Introduction. In *Viral Dramaturgies: HIV and AIDS in Performance in the Twenty-First Century*, ed. Alyson Campbell and Dirk Gindt, 343–365. Springer International Publishing.

Campbell, Alyson, and Jonathan Graffam. 2018. Blood, Shame, Resilience and Hope: Indigenous Theatre Maker Jacob Boehme's *Blood on the Dance Floor*. In *Viral Dramaturgies: HIV and AIDS in Performance in the Twenty-First Century*, ed. Alyson Campbell and Dirk Gindt, 343–365. Springer International Publishing.

Gee, Graham, Pat Dudgeon, Clinton Schultz, Amanda Hart, and Kerrie Kelly. 2014. Aboriginal and Torres Strait Islander Social and Emotional Wellbeing. In *Working Together: Aboriginal and Torres Strait Islander Mental Health and Wellbeing Principles and Practice*, ed. Pat Dudgeon, Helen Milroy, and Roz Walker, 55–68. Canberra: Commonwealth of Australia.

Keating, Clare. 2009. *'Chopped Liver' Evaluation Report*. Effective Change Pty Ltd. Melbourne: Ilbijerri Theatre Company. Supplied.

Low, Katharine E. 2017. Understanding Health, Wellbeing, the Millennium Development Goals and Health Inequities. In *Applied Theatre: Performing Health and Wellbeing*, ed. Veronica Baxter and Katharine E. Low, 11–40. London: Bloomsbury Methuen Drama. https://doi.org/10.5040/9781472584601.ch-001.

———. 2020. *Applied Theatre and Sexual Health Communication: Apertures of Possibility*. London: Palgrave Macmillan.

Prendergast, Monica, and Juliana Saxton, eds. 2016. *Applied Theatre: International Case Studies and Challenges for Practice (Second Edition)*. Intellect Books.

Scar Trees. 2019. By Declan Furber Gillick. Adapted by Kamarra Bell-Wykes. Directed by Kamarra Bell-Wykes. Premiered at Northcote Town Hall, Melbourne, Victoria, October 28.

Viral – Are You the Cure? 2018. By Maryann Sam. Directed by Kamarra Bell-Wykes. Various sites throughout Victoria, 2018–2019.

Wells, Trish. 2013. Insights into Approaching Sexual Health Education Through Applied Theatre Methodology. *Applied Theatre Research* 1 (2): 203–215. https://doi.org/10.1386/atr.1.2.203_1.

Welsh, Blayne. 2018. The Hepatitis C Trilogy: A Case for Indigenous Theatre as a Contemporary Manifestation of Traditional Healing Business. *Australasian Drama Studies* 73: 20–41. https://search.informit.org/doi/abs/10.3316/ielapa.146479491877297.

CHAPTER 7

Conclusion

Abstract This chapter concludes our study of health education works produced by Australia's Ilbijerri Theatre Company and led by Yuggera and Butchulla theatre maker Kamarra Bell-Wykes from 2006 to 2019. We draw together the findings to conclude that the works *Chopped Liver*, *Body Armour*, *Viral – Are You the Cure?*, *North West of Nowhere*, and *Scar Trees* represent a significant and innovative contribution to both First Nations contemporary theatre and applied theatre for health education and equity. Looking back on this important body of work has also informed the development of future projects for Kamarra, including the most recent work, *The Score*, which addresses sexual health for young Aboriginal and Torres Strait Islander peoples through a community-engaged, participatory model. We conclude by acknowledging the creative teams who contributed to these works over 13 years, recognising that the success of these works was built on their talent, dedication, and commitment.

Keywords First Nations theatre • Theatre in education • Applied theatre • Arts and health • Theatre for health education

We embarked on this project with the goal of critically examining the health education works produced by Ilbijerri Theatre Company and led by Kamarra between 2006 and 2019, while also documenting and honouring

S. Woodland, K. Bell-Wykes, *First Nations Australian Theatre for Health Equity*, https://doi.org/10.1007/978-3-031-65506-7_7

the legacy of this important yet underreported body of work. Reaching over 26,000 audience members and garnering numerous awards, the works have contributed to the continuing tradition of cultural storytelling, performance, education, and healing ceremonies practised by Aboriginal and Torres Strait Islander communities for millennia. In bridging contemporary Australian First Nations performance with applied theatre, an analysis of the plays offers valuable insights into global health promotion and education through theatre from a unique perspective. Throughout the book, we have examined the creative processes, cultural significance, and educational impact of these works, situating them within a holistic framework that extends beyond health messaging and social impact and into dramaturgies community wellbeing, strength, and resistance.

Summary of Findings

We acknowledge that this study had some limitations, given that we commenced work in 2020, long after the performances under examination had finished touring. This meant relying on the recollections of creative team members, as well as incomplete archival documentation and incomplete audience survey data that was collected with a different purpose in mind (i.e., to demonstrate the short-term impact on audiences to funders and stakeholders). Nevertheless, we identified three central themes within the data that, although separated here, interact with each other in a holistic sense to tell the story of a powerful body of culturally led, community-engaged performance practice—one that offers significant lessons regarding arts-led approaches to health and wellbeing, applicable not only to First Nations communities but also to a broader context.

1. **Culturally led, culturally safe performance making**

The findings emphasise the importance of First Nations cultural leadership throughout the creative process, privileging diverse lived experiences and foregrounding community engagement and cultural safety for creative teams and audiences. This approach was seen as foundational to working ethically and relationally, achieving educational objectives, and advancing contemporary First Nations theatre as characterised by themes of community wellbeing, strength, and resistance.

2. **The 'gripping dramatic yarn'**

The works are framed as captivating narratives that incorporated cultural storytelling, authenticity, engaging characters, humour, and strong performances. They artfully blended entertainment and education, engaging audiences and conveying health-related messages, while also speaking to the wider social and political contexts and empowering First Nations audiences through reflecting the strengths, complexity, and diversity of their communities.

3. **Stigma-free spaces for healing, empowerment, and self-determination**

The works facilitated culturally safe spaces for conveying health messages, challenging stigma, and fostering community empowerment and capacity building. They went beyond individualised notions of behaviour change to embrace a holistic notion of wellbeing that includes resistance to colonial structures and self-determination. This contributed to personal growth and transformation among various stakeholders, including audience members, health professionals, performers, and creatives. We suggest that this approach, in some cases, contributed in a holistic sense to community wellbeing.

Key Learnings

The findings summarised above can be seen as foundational principles to adopt in theatre for health education projects in First Nations communities—perhaps translatable to other arts-led approaches and community contexts as well. We do acknowledge, however, that some key learnings have also emerged around how to promote the long-term sustainability for programs and to further strengthen and extend their impacts in communities.

1. **Deeper and more extensive community engagement in the lead up to touring**

The experience of teams turning up at a venue only to find one or two people in the audience illustrates the need for meaningful and sustained community consultation and engagement at every stage of the project. This includes finding a range of different people in the community from the grassroots level to community-controlled organisations and local Elders so that the project is not dependent on the recommendations of just one person. In a sector that is known for its high turnover and overworked staff, this will also help to mitigate against projects failing if that one key person is away or has moved on by the time of delivery. This may be supported by theatre companies employing producers who have interest and experience in community development practices. Nevertheless, we acknowledge the challenges of working to develop and sustain relationships over the longer term, given that this is often in tension with the demands of mainstream Western health promotion delivery and funding models. However, by continuing to foreground the importance of this approach through studies such as these, we hope that it may be possible to educate mainstream partners and funders to expect that this is a legitimate and vital process that will improve sustainable impacts and outcomes.

2. **Working productively with health partners and stakeholders**

Building on the previous point, we suggest that cultivating relationships with mainstream health partners, funders, and stakeholders over time will strengthen opportunities for mutual trust and respect that can lead to stronger artistic freedom. Nevertheless, it is vital for artists to maintain a strong stance when it comes to artistic decision-making and to ensure that the aesthetic and performative elements of a work are not compromised by the need to include specific health messages or scenarios. The artistry demonstrated by the creative teams in the works discussed in this volume suggests that artists need to feel confident in their capacity to make highly engaging educational theatre works and to become leaders in using the arts for social change (as opposed to following the whims and trends of policy and practice in health or other social sectors). This of course extends to standing firm on matters of First Nations cultural leadership and knowledge transmission, which must not be subsumed by mainstream institutional methods and priorities.

3. **Stronger cultural safety protocols for creative teams**

While we identified a strong sense of cultural safety and support for creative teams in many of these works, this was not necessarily consistent across all projects and was dependent on the skills and abilities of those charged with leading or holding space at the time. We recognise the need for theatre companies to adopt detailed and consistent protocols for supporting First Nations artists to deliver this kind of work in communities, where the 'colonial load' potentially extends beyond telling difficult stories and into a deeper sense of responsibility to engage ethically with audiences. This could be achieved through policy making and staff training at the organisational level, perhaps to place a higher value on this kind of work that can often be sidelined in favour of the mainstage, as well as developing consistent practices for briefing, debriefing, and supervision for teams at all stages. Attending to the wellbeing of creative teams will enable them to focus on doing their best work without becoming exhausted or burnt out.

4. **Strengthening community engagement and participation in the plays**

The lessons from *Viral* point towards the power of conducting workshops with communities that directly inform characters and storylines. This strengthens empowerment and engagement for audiences who recognise themselves in the work and can feel a sense of pride and ownership. It also deepens the authenticity of stories and characters for a wider audience, who see themselves reflected in the work. The workshops themselves serve as powerful, reciprocal sites for learning and knowledge transmission, strengthening cultural practices and collaborations towards community wellbeing. The inclusion of non-professional community members in the cast (as in the case of Shannon Hood) brought home the power of presenting an accessible peer on stage who can offer inspiration and aspiration to audiences who may never have previously imagined themselves in such a highly skilled performance and leadership role.

Looking Forward: *The Score*

As signalled throughout this book, the study's findings have greatly informed how Kamarra now approaches the work, which has evolved over the course of her engagement with the health education works since 2006. While the health education performances discussed here were successful on many levels, they largely followed a conventional approach—relying on commissioned playwrights, professional actors, and community touring. Through experimenting with community-engaged approaches to making works such as *Scar Trees* and *Viral*, Kamarra now recognises the value of intentionally building works with community from the ground up.

Particularly through *Viral*, where the workshops in prisons informed the development of the performance, the return to prison resulted in deeper engagement from those men who had participated in the workshops, as did the inclusion of Shannon Hood in the cast, who had some aligned experiences and connections to the incarcerated community. This "full circle" approach has led to the development of the new model, *The Score*, focused on sexual health and respectful relationships for Aboriginal and Torres Strait Islander young people, which, through its reimagining of how to approach health education through theatre, has resulted in the creation of a new participatory model. The model draws together some similar performance aesthetics from the previous works and merges them intentionally with approaches from theatre in education and participatory theatre, contrasting with the traditional "fly in-fly out" method and serving as a promising direction for achieving lasting health and wellbeing outcomes.

As discussed earlier, Victoria's Department of Health funded *The Score* to address its concerns around the persistent "gap" between sexual health outcomes for First Nations communities and the broader population. The Department was broadly supportive of taking a new approach and could see the merit in working towards more sustainable impacts in communities via deeper participation and engagement. A reference group consisting of sexual health experts from the Victorian Aboriginal Community Controlled Organisation (VACCHO) and Thorne Harbour Health again were invited to contribute their specialist knowledge. With her expertise in applied and educational theatre, Sarah brought the University of Melbourne's Faculty of Fine Arts and Music on board as a partner, securing funding from the Australian Institute for Aboriginal and Torres Strait Islander Studies (AIATSIS) to develop the model, research the outcomes, and build capacity in communities through professional development training so that the theatre-based approaches could be taken up and used to address local health and wellbeing concerns.

The Score commenced production in 2021 where an ensemble of six young performers and the creative team worked with theatre maker Stefo Nantsou from Zeal Theatre Company to devise a high-energy performance that would surface the issues for a young audience. Pongjit Saphakhun and Richard Barber from Free Theatre contributed their insights from delivering their brand of "dialogue theatre" in communities in Australia, Thailand, and Myanmar. For Kamarra, who places a high value on continuous learning and creative collaborations with other artists and practitioners, the new model has provided an opportunity for an interdisciplinary team to form around the work, strengthening its performative outcomes and theoretical rigour. Working through three iterations of development, the team established a model that consists of four phases and is, at the time of writing, currently being rolled out in Victorian metropolitan and regional communities:

Phase one: The "kick-off" performance of *The Score*: "A short play with big energy about footy, friends, dancing and hookups" (Ilbijerri n.d.) follows the adventures of two protagonists, Sam and Billy, as they navigate the after-party of the local football carnival. Running for only seven minutes, the play is facilitated by the "Coach" who acts as an intermediary between the action on stage and the audience, facilitating dialogue around the issues raised. The kick-off performance serves as a hook to draw in young people so that they then hopefully sign up for the residency that follows.

Phase two: A workshop residency that invites young people in the community to unpack the issues surfaced by the kick-off performance through yarning, drama, and experiential methods. Through the residency, young people are also rehearsed into *The Score* and invited to contribute their own characters, perspectives, and approaches to the performance. Some of this work takes place through a culturally safe frame of gendered yarning circles, where men's business, women's business, and "rainbow" (or gender diverse) business can be discussed in a closed circle before returning to the whole group.

Phase three: A "grand final" performance where the young participants perform *The Score* alongside the ensemble to an audience of invited friends, family, and community members. This is again facilitated by the Coach, who invites responses from the audience around the barriers and enablers to sexual health in their community.

Phase four: Members of the team and ensemble train up local professionals in health and social care to use the theatre-based and experiential methods featured in the model and adapt them for their own needs and purposes.

The Score kick-off performance retained several of the aesthetic elements that were successful in previous health education performances, such as the 'world' of the regional footy carnival and after party that is highly recognisable to many First Nations communities; strong, identifiable character archetypes of Brotha-Boys, Sista-Gals, Aunties, and Uncles, which place the responsibility for young people's sexual health beyond the individual and into the community's hands; humour and playfulness in the dialogue; and high energy music and choreography that includes a culturally informed 'courtship dance' that fuses with contemporary dance floor energy. These elements contribute to depicting the issue (sexual health) as grounded in fun and joy rather than shame and stigma and serve to demonstrate the complexity of making healthy choices in the context of a highly charged social moment. The ensemble of six performers plays across gender throughout, with the Brotha-Boy and Sista-Gal characters providing the audience-participants an opportunity to embrace queer representation within the world of the play through a cultural frame (if applicable to the group).[1] The protagonists, Sam and Billy, serve a similar function to those found in most educational theatre that draws from Theatre of the Oppressed (Boal 1985), enabling the audience-participants to project their own experiences onto them and invest in their choices and decisions through the protection of the fiction. The "Coach" character draws heavily on the legacy of the Joker in Boal's Forum Theatre, facilitating dialogue with the audience that unpacks the issue and delves into its complexities and nuances.

The Score model also embraces and extends some of the principles that have underpinned the health education works throughout, for example, by adopting a holistic approach to health and wellbeing that moves beyond individual behaviours and aims to contribute to empowerment, self-determination, and community wellbeing. The model extends the community engagement processes used in productions like *Viral* to adopt a place-based approach centring First Nations knowledges, young people's experiences and stories, and those of their communities. This includes identifying localised risk and protective factors to sexual health and healthy relationships and working to create stronger links with local health and youth services and organisations. With funding from AIATSIS, we have also had the opportunity to engage in a more intentional, holistic research process from the start that centres culturally informed methods such as yarning and performance (Woodland et al. 2023). A key part of this design is the capacity-building phase, which aims to further strengthen outcomes in communities. This research is still underway; however, early indications suggest that moving to a participatory model has successfully engaged young people in culturally safe, stigma-free yarning around sexual health and healthy relationships, has increased skills and capacities in performance and community engagement for *The Score* ensemble, and has deepened

[1] In Aboriginal and Torres Strait Islander cultures, these interchangeable relationship terms can refer to a close friend/family member or someone who identifies as LGBTIAQ+, depending on the context (Farrell 2015).

the engagement and investment from community members in both the creative process and the health issues being explored, which we hope will lead to more meaningful and lasting impacts.

Several of our interview subjects for this study into the health education works from 2006 to 2019 were keen to see the work develop in this direction, agreeing that it would be a positive step in evolving the work. Melodie Reynolds-Diarra saw it as a natural return to more traditional kinds of storytelling:

> It's not any one person's story then because it's many people's stories and, as soon as you've put more voices in there, more ears are going to listen. … In giving the voice to the people - the community, as soon as you're getting a voice, it's like learning how to use a muscle. So, if you haven't had the chance to use that muscle and you haven't had a voice for so long, you need to be taught how to do that once again. … It feels like that natural thing of, you know, all sitting around the fire and all having turns to talk. (Interview, 2021)

Isaac Drandic highlighted the capacity-building potential of such a model, "You're actually kind of leaving the communities with something, with some kind of valuable skills and valuable tools that they can then kind of continue to use long after the circus has left town" (interview, 2021). Nazaree Dickerson also spoke about how many projects are "flash in the pan" and that a model like this has the potential to leave behind a legacy. Nazaree went on to describe the potential for empowering communities through this approach: "A show that they've seen is great, but if there's a show they've been in and it's their story or their mob's story, that's even better" (interview, 2021). Similarly, Isaac suggested, "To be … in control of your own stories and to have input into your own stories is just such a kind of important part of growing confidence and feeling valued and valuable and creating theatre … it's a powerful practice." Shannon Hood, the only inexperienced community performer to be cast in this body of work, suggested, "I think creating something like that and then if you were to go out and perform it, I think I'd be a lot more passionate about it" (interview, 2021). This has been borne out by some of the early feedback we have received from young people participating in *The Score* residencies so far, who have expressed how the work clearly connects to them because it represents "real" life and integrates their own stories and perspectives.

Conclusion

Throughout this book, we have articulated the creative processes used to develop the health education works, explored their cultural, aesthetic, and educational dimensions, and assessed their impact on creatives, audiences, and communities. In examining the work from a unique First Nations Australian perspective, we have gained invaluable insights that might contribute to understanding theatre for health education and promotion globally, where the liveness, immediacy, and interactivity of such performances continue to be valued as an alternative to more traditional 'dry' approaches. Further, our findings provide a set of principles and approaches that practitioners might adopt in working towards the artful integration of education and performance aesthetics, advancing the notion of applied or educational theatre as a legitimate art form in its own right. Beyond their focus on health messaging and education, we argue that through considered practices of culturally led, culturally safe, community-informed performance making, the works assert sovereignty for Aboriginal and Torres Strait Islander peoples over the structures and institutions that inform such projects, contributing to decolonising health education, health promotion, community development, research, and theatre. By situating the works within the canon of contemporary First Nations theatre in Australia, we argue that they contribute to dramaturgies of community wellbeing, strength, and resistance that are integral to Aboriginal and Torres Strait Islander self-determination and survival in this country.

There exists a strong legacy of leadership and creative contributions within Ilbijerri and its partners and stakeholders that have supported the health education works in their Social Impact stream since 2006. Successive members of Ilbijerri's leadership and Board have recognised the importance and value of these works and participated in their artistic development. In addition, each of the works has had a team of key creative and production personnel and government and non-government partners whose talent, dedication, and commitment have been integral to the works' success. We would like to conclude our study by acknowledging them here and thanking all who have participated in creating this powerful body of work.

Production Teams

Chopped Liver (2006–2009)

Writer: Kamarra Bell-Wykes
Dramaturg: John Romeril

Director: Kylie Belling (2006–2007), Rachael Maza (2008)
Designer: Destiny Deacon, Virginia Fraser (2006–2007)
Sound Designer: Steph O'Hara (2006–2009)
Visual Designer: Destiny Deacon, Virginia Fraser
Tour Manager: Lisa Maza (2007–2008), Lisa Parris (2009)
Stage Manager: PJ Rosas (2006–2008), Lionel Austin (2006, 2009)
Performers: Isaac Drandic (2006–2009), Melodie Reynolds (2006–2008), Nikki Ashby (2008), Cy Fahey (2009)

Chopped Liver **(2017)**

Writer and Director: Kamarra Bell-Wykes
Dramaturg: John Romeril
Set and Costume Designer: Darryl Cordell
Sound Designer: Richie Hallal
Tour Facilitator: Richie Hallal
Stage Manager: Ari Maza Long
Performers: Gregory J Fryer and Nazaree Dickerson

Body Armour **(2010–2013)**

Writer: Kamarra Bell-Wykes
Dramaturge: John Romeril
Director: Margaret Harvey
Set and Costume Designer: Alison Ross
Sound Designer: Anna Liebzeit
Tour and Stage Manager: Bronwyn Dunstan (2010), Caitlin Chessell (2011), Bec Cooen (2012), Jessica Smithett (2013).
Performers: LeRoy Parsons (2010–2013), Maurial Spearim (2010–2013), Sandy Greenwood (2010, 2011, 2013), Uraine Mastrosavas (2012).

Viral – Are You the Cure? **(2018–2019)**

Writer: Maryanne Sam
Director/Dramaturg: Kamarra Bell-Wykes (2018–2019)
Choreographer: Carly Sheppard
Set and Sound Designer: small sound
Costume Designer: Jacinta Keefe
Producer: Davey Thompson (2018), Lisa Parris (2019)
Associate Producer: Emily Anypa Butcher

Production Manager: Caleb Thaiday (2018–2019)
Stage Manager: Mary Quinsacara (2018)
Community Consultation Facilitators: Shiralee Hood and Kamarra Bell-Wykes (2018)
Facilitation Consultation and Training: Free Theatre (2018)
Community Engagement Manager: Richie Hallal (2019)
Performers: Laila Thaker (2018), Jesse Butler (2018–2019), Blayne Welsh (2018–2019), Nikita Tabuteau (2019), Shannon Hood (2019).

***North West of Nowhere* (2014–2016)**

Writer: Kamarra Bell-Wykes
Dramaturg: John Romeril
Director: Rachael Maza (2014–2015), Eva Grace Mullaley (2016)
Set and Costume Designer: Emily Barrie
Sound Designer and Musician: James Henry
Choreography: Carly Sheppard
Tour and Stage Manager: Ruth Maloney (2014), Brock Brocklesby (2015–2016)
Performers: Shaynee Brayshaw (2014), Carly Sheppard (2015), Ian Michaels (2014–2015), James Henry (2014–2015), Jack Sheppard (2016), Brandi Nelson (2016), Jesse Butler (2016).
Health Worker: Tarneen Onus-Williams (2015), Lenka Vanderboom (2016)

***Scar Trees* (2019)**

Writer: Declan Furber-Gillick
Dramaturg and Director: Kamarra Bell-Wykes
Performers: Dion Williams, Maurial Spearim, Racheal Oak Butler
Set and Sound Design: small sound
Costume Consultant: Jacinta Keefe
Social Impact Producer: Lisa Parris
Associate Producer: J-Maine Beezley
Stage and Production Manager: Brock Brocklesby
Family Violence Support Coordinator: Nazaree Dickerson

***The Score* (2021–)**

Ensemble Members: Baydon Clayton (2021), Nazaree Dickerson (2021–2022), Axel Garay (2021), Monique Grbec (2021), Lisa Maza (2021), Jerrika Pevitt (2021), Andrew (Balaneba) Toby (2021), Zerene

Webster (2021–2023), Zane Webster (2022–2023), Zach Blampied (2023), Kimmie Lovegrove (2023), Corey Saylor-Brunskill (2022–2023), Taeg Twist (2023).

Devising Facilitators: Stefo Nantsou, Kamarra Bell-Wykes, Free Theatre

Social Impact Producer: Kim Bennett (2020–2021), Laura Harris (2022)

Community Coordinator: Della Bedford

Associate Producer: Lauren Sheree (2020–2021); Theo Cassady (2022)

Stage/Tour Manager: Jenny Le (2023)

Researcher and Facilitator: Sarah Woodland

Partners and Supporters

Aboriginal Health and Medical Research Council (AHMRC)
Aboriginal Health Council of South Australia
Australian Institute of Aboriginal and Torres Strait Islander Studies (AIATSIS)
Australian Research Centre in Sex, Health and Society—La Trobe University
Bendigo and District Aboriginal Co-operative (BDAC)
Bunjilwarra Koori Youth Alcohol and Drug Healing Service
Centre for Excellence in Rural Sexual Health (CERSH)
Creative Victoria
Dandenong and District Aboriginal Cooperative
Department of Health and Human Services (DHHS)
Department of Justice and Community Safety, Victoria
Family Planning Victoria
Gandel Foundation
Helen Macpherson Smith Trust
Hepatitis New South Wales
Hepatitis South Australia
Hepatitis Victoria
Hepatitis Western Australia
Institute of Koori Education—Deakin University (NIKERI)
Korin Gamadji Institute
Lord Mayor's Charitable Foundation, Melbourne
Odyssey House
Rumbalara Aboriginal Co-operative
Star Health
University of Melbourne
Victorian Aboriginal Child Care Agency (VACCA)
Victorian Aboriginal Community Controlled Health Organisation (VACCHO)
Victorian Aboriginal Health Service (VAHS)
Victorian AIDS Council (Thorne Harbour Health)
Victorian Health Promotion Foundation (VicHealth)
Women's Health West

References

Boal, Augusto. 1985. Theatre of the Oppressed. Translated by A. Charles, and Maria-Odilia Leal McBride. New York: Theatre Communications Group.

Farrell, Andrew. 2015. Can You See Me? Queer Margins in Aboriginal Communities. *Journal of Global Indigeneity* 1 (1): 1–4. https://www.jstor.org/stable/48717628.

Ilbijerri Theatre Company. n.d. *The Score*. Accessed September 23, 2023. https://www.ilbijerri.com.au/event/thescore/

Scar Trees. 2019. By Declan Furber Gillick. Adapted by Kamarra Bell-Wykes. Directed by Kamarra Bell-Wykes. Premiered at Northcote Town Hall, Melbourne, Victoria, October 28, 2019.

Woodland, Sarah, Kamarra Bell-Wykes, and Carissa Lee Godwin. 2023. Yarning Up Relations: Enacting a Relational Ethics in Cross-Cultural Research-Based Theater. *Qualitative Inquiry* 29 (2): 393–402. https://doi.org/10.1177/10778004221099561.

Afterword

There is no doubt this book will be an invaluable resource, inspiring and informing the next generation of Blak Theatre makers.

I was a child when the first Blak Theatre company was established—born out of the Black Power and Self-Determination movement in the early 1970s—finally, we had a platform for our voices, our stories, and for our mob, unapologetically political. Like the guitar—'theatre' is a tool that we quickly appropriated and mastered, though the process of decolonising/indigenising these tools continues.

Kamarra Bell-Wykes is one of those artists leading the charge. I've watched and worked with Kamarra for over 20 years now and have long been in awe of and inspired by her uncompromising cultural and artistic integrity and talent. Every new project has been an opportunity to further develop and deepen her practice through the practical application of a methodology based on Blak ways of working; from the process (how we make the work) to deepening the relationship/engagement with audience/community through to the sector itself and how the work is funded.

More recently, I've had the honour of meeting Sarah Woodland whose extensive experience in "applied theatre" and equally sharp intellect and

S. Woodland, K. Bell-Wykes, *First Nations Australian Theatre for Health Equity*, https://doi.org/10.1007/978-3-031-65506-7

passion and belief that theatre is a powerful tool for change has made her the perfect collaborator with Kamarra and made possible in this brilliant resource.

This work gives me great hope for what's to come—watch this space.

ILBIJERRI Theatre Company
Melbourne, VIC, Australia
September 2023

Rachael Maza AM

Index[1]

A

B

C

[1] Note: Page numbers followed by 'n' refer to notes.

S. Woodland, K. Bell-Wykes, *First Nations Australian Theatre for Health Equity*, https://doi.org/10.1007/978-3-031-65506-7